Narrative Based Medicine

To our patients and their families and carers, whose stories of illness, healing, coping and dying have been the inspiration for this book.

Narrative Based Medicine

Dialogue and discourse in clinical practice

Edited by

TRISHA GREENHALGH
General Practitioner and Senior Lecturer, Department of Primary Care and Population Sciences, University College London and Royal Free Hospital Schools of Medicine, Whittington Hospital, London, UK

BRIAN HURWITZ
General Practitioner and Senior Lecturer, Department of General Practice and Primary Health Care, Imperial College School of Medicine, London, UK

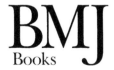

© BMJ Books 1998
BMJ Books is an imprint of the BMJ Publishing Group

First published in 1998
Reprinted 1999
by BMJ Books, BMA House, Tavistock Square,
London WC1H 9JR

British Library Cataloguing in Publication Data

A catalogue record for this book is available from the British Library

ISBN 0-7279-1223-2

Typeset by Apek Typesetters, Nailsea, Bristol
Printed and bound by Latimer Trend, Plymouth.

Contents

Contributors

Donald Bateman left school in Leeds at 14 and became a printer's apprentice. All his education has been via the Further Education part-time route and at retirement he was Head of Faculty at Brunel College. He spent 10 years as Chair of governors of that college and he is now a governor of the City of Bristol College. He is now a print consultant.

Sir Richard Bayliss is a physician and endocrinologist whose many past academic distinctions include Dean of Westminster Hospital Medical School (1960–65) and President of the Association of Physicians; he is now semi-retired and practices as a thyroidologist.

Gillie Bolton is Research Fellow in Medical Humanities at Sheffield University Institute of General Practice. Her book, *The therapeutic potential of creative writing: writing myself*, will be published by Jessica Kingsley Publishers in September 1998; her research is also into writing as a reflective practitioner.

Howard Brody is a family physician and professor of medical ethics at Michigan State University, East Lansing, Michigan, USA. He is the author of *Stories of sickness* and *The healer's power*, as well as papers on narrative ethics.

Anna Donald is a clinical lecturer in epidemiology and public health at University College London. She studies the effects of poverty on health and teaches epidemiology and health policy to masters and undergraduate students.

James Owen Drife is a professor of obstetrics and gynaecology at the University of Leeds and a consultant at Leeds General Infirmary. He is Clinical Chairman of the UK Confidential Enquiry into Maternal Deaths.

Glyn Elwyn works as a general practitioner at the Ely Bridge Surgery in Cardiff and is a senior lecturer in general practice at the University of Wales College of Medicine. His research interests include sharing decisions with patients, the contextual aspects of health care and evidence based practice – and the interface between these areas.

Paramjit Gill is a senior lecturer in primary care at the University of Birmingham.

Stephen Jay Gould teaches Geology, Biology and History of Science at Harvard University where he holds chairs in Zoology and Geology. He is Curator of Invertebrate Palaeontology at the University's Museum of Comparative Zoology, and has written many books about evolutionary biology, including *Ever since Darwin, The panda's thumb, Wonderful life, Eight little piggies, The mismeasure of man, Dinosaur in a haystack*, and *Life's grandeur*.

Trisha Greenhalgh is a part-time general practitioner in north London and a senior lecturer in primary care at the Royal Free and University College London Medical Schools where she is also Director of the Unit for Evidence Based Practice and Policy. Her research interests include the use of narrative in the education of patients and health professionals and the theoretical basis of evidence based medicine.

Richard Gwyn is research co-ordinator at the Health Communication Research Centre, Cardiff University, where he teaches an undergraduate module in "Health Communication". He is currently writing a book on the discourses of health and illness, which emphasises the narrative foundation of illness experience.

Iona Heath is a general practitioner in North London and author of *The mystery of general practice*.

Stuart Hogarth studied history at the University of North London before going on to study the history of science and medicine at the Wellcome Institute and Imperial College. He is currently completing a PhD on working-class attitudes to health and sickness in 19th century Britain.

Jeremy Holmes is a consultant psychotherapist in North Devon, and chair of the Psychotherapy Faculty of the Royal College of Psychiatrists. His most recent book is *Healing stories: narrative in psychiatry and psychotherapy* (with G Roberts; Oxford University Press, 1998). His interests include poetry, politics, and personality disorders.

Anne Hudson Jones is Professor of Literature and Medicine in the Institute for the Medical Humanities of The University of Texas Medical Branch at Galveston, where she teaches courses in literature and medicine and in medical ethics. A founding editor of *Literature and Medicine*, she was the journal's editor-in-chief for more than 10 years. She has recently published articles on narrative ethics in *The Journal of Medicine and Philosophy* and *The Lancet*.

Brian Hurwitz is a part-time general practitioner in central London and a senior lecturer in general practice and primary care at the Imperial College School of Medicine in west London. His research interests include improving the primary care of the patients with chronic disease, medical ethics, law, and narrative; his book *Clinical guidelines and the law* was published in 1998 (Radcliffe Medical Press).

Steve Kay is a senior lecturer in Computer Science at the University of Manchester; co-founder and leader of the research group in Medical Informatics. His research interests relate to clinical record systems and the study of narratology. In this context, he leads a European project on the Electronic Health Care Record Architecture, using concepts derived from studies of narrative structure to inform the technical standard being developed.

John Launer is a general practitioner in Edmonton, north London, and is also Senior Clinical Lecturer in General Practice at the Tavistock Clinic. He is a family therapist and GP educator, with a special interest in the application of family therapy, ideas and skills to everyday general practice.

Jane Macnaughton is a part-time GP and a lecturer in the Department of General Practice at Glasgow University. Prior to studying medicine she read literature and is currently working for a PhD on evidence and insight in the practice of medicine.

Marshall Marinker has been a GP, a professor of General Practice, and acts as an independent consultant on medical education, health care research and policy.

Lara Marks has a Wellcome Award in the History of Medicine based at Imperial College. She has published a number of books and articles on the history of maternal and child health and questions of ethnicity and health, and is currently completing a book on the history of the contraceptive pill (Yale University Press).

Robert McCrum is literary editor of the Observer newspaper. His book *My year off: rediscovering life after a stroke*, was published by Picador in 1988.

Ian Purves is a GP by training and is now Head of the Sowerby Centre for Health Informatics at Newcastle University. He has contributed widely to health informatics and General Practice literature on many diverse subjects, his interest in naratology came from trying to understand and develop the health record.

Stephen Rachman holds a PhD in American Studies from Yale University. He teaches courses in literature and medicine at Michigan State University. He is the co-editor of *The American face of Edgar Allan Poe* and the forthcoming study *Cultural pathology: disease and literature in 19th century America*.

Ruth Richardson is a Wellcome Research Fellow in the History of Medicine at the Department of Anatomy, University College London. Her book, *Death, dissection and the destitute* (Penguin, 1989) traces the sources of corpses for anatomy from the Renaissance to the present day. The staff of medical museums in Britain and Europe are thanked for their kindness to her during the research which led to the writing of *Organ music*.

P Anne Scott is a senior lecturer in Nursing and Ethics at the Department of Nursing and Midwifery at the University of Stirling. Her research interests are in the area of health care ethics and medical humanities, with particular interests in virtue theory and the role of the moral imagination.

Vieda Skultans is a social anthropologist at the University of Bristol. She teaches on the Human Basis of Medicine course. Her book *The testimony of lives: narrative and memory in post-Soviet Latvia* was published by Routledge in 1997.

Harriet Squier is a family practitioner and Associate Adjunct Professor at the Centre for Ethics and Humanities in the Life Sciences at Michigan State University. She has published on literature and medicine and the doctor–patient relationship, and has designed innovative medical school curricula on the doctor–patient relationship, family practice, and literature and medicine including electives on women and medicine, death and dying, minorities and medicine, and the meaning of illness.

Henerietta Weinbren is an academic training fellow at the Department of Primary Care and Population Sciences, University College London.

Foreword

Why should health professionals care about what is in this book? Narrative is important in medicine because it performs a great many bridging functions.

First, telling any narrative in any setting is a bridging performance. Most obviously, it connects the teller and the listener. One cannot begin mentally to construct a narrative without immediately (if implicitly) imagining an audience. The more one studies narrative, the more one realises how very complex this bridge between teller and listener actually is. For instance, the act of telling a story to the listener changes the story. Just as one cannot step into the same river twice, the narrator cannot ever tell exactly the "same" narrative again. Telling a story and repeating a story are two subtly different forms of action. On the listener's side, none of us ever truly "hears" a story exactly as it is told by the narrator. Each story inevitably has gaps of meaning and significance, and we fill in these gaps as we imagine the world to be and as we imagine the teller intended. Thus, rather than hear a story, it is rather more accurate to say that we construct for ourselves a story about what we think we are hearing. The bridge between teller and listener of a story turns out not only to carry traffic in both directions, but to carry multiple levels of traffic as well.

Second, Anne Hudson Jones, as quoted in Chapter 9, speaks of how "doctors travel back and forth across the bridge, taking the patient's story of illness to be ... retold in the form of a case history." Here the simple metaphor of the bridge threatens to obscure some of the most difficult and perplexing issues in medical practice. The issue, at its core, is elegantly summarised by Platt, quoted in Chapter 1: "The first staggering fact about medical education is that after two and a half years of being taught on the assumption that everyone is the same the student has to find out for himself that everyone is different, which is what his experience has taught him since infancy." Some of medicine works extremely well precisely because it treats people as being all the same; and some of medicine works very well because it treats people as all being different. Physicians must constantly juggle these two ways of seeing their patients.

To deal with the part of medicine which treats everyone as the same, we must extract the narrative from the patient and recast it as a "case history" or as a medicalised retelling of the story. If we do not do this we can never bring to the patient the undoubted benefits of modern medical science. If we do only this, we dehumanise the patient, fail to address him or her as an individual, and ultimately may very well increase the patient's suffering. As Jones insists, we must take the case history back across the bridge and help the patient to link it effectively with the life-experience narrative he or she is trying to construct to make sense of the illness. Clinical encounters being what they are, this is seldom a simple, two-stage process. Throughout an encounter, the narrative may travel back and forth across the bridge, to be modified in turn on the medical and on the lived-experience side, in a sort of shuttle diplomacy that might make achieving peace in the Middle East look simple by comparison.

Of the two sides of this bridge, modern biomedicine has most recently tended to neglect the patient or the lived-experience side; and calls to "humanise" medicine demand that we redress this imbalance. But that does not mean that we can afford to neglect the physician's side. Kathryn Montgomery Hunter, whose seminal work *Doctors' Stories* has influenced many of the following selections, makes clear that medical thinking is basically a form of narrative work. The chapters in this book allow us to see both sides of the bridge with equal vividness.

Finally, as this volume attests, the study of narrative builds bridges among the various disciplines that all have something interesting and important to say about medical practice, research, and education. Since narrative in medicine began to receive attention in the mid-1980s, we have seen dialogue emerge among physicians, nurses, literary critics, social scientists, linguistic analysts, information theorists, philosophers, and many other scholars and practitioners. "The story" turns out to be an especially vital point of intersection among work in many different fields; and becoming sensitised to its own dependence on narrative has opened medicine to useful input from all of these fields. In a time of uncertainty and turmoil in medical practice and organisation, such a broad base of interdisciplinary dialogue cannot help but be salutary.

This collection both incorporates the bridges that have been built, or are now under construction, and tells us where we need more and better bridges in the future. Since most people would have said as recently as 1982 that stories are an unimportant and uninteresting feature of medicine, progress has been nothing short of astounding.

Howard Brody
Centre for Ethics and Humanities in the Life Sciences
Michigan State University
USA

Acknowledgments

This book contains the writings, drawings and medical details of numerous patients who have generously shared their most intimate experiences of illness and suffering. We thank them sincerely, and we share their hope that their personal stories will help improve public and professional understanding of what it means to be ill, and thereby enhance the quality of care that health professionals provide to patients.

The production of any multi-author textbook is a major collaborative venture between editors, chapter authors, referees, and publisher. We thank our 27 co-authors for their diverse contributions, and for their patience and perseverance when we requested yet another addition or amendment to their work. We thank, especially, those authors who acted as sounding boards for our own thoughts and as anonymous peer reviewers for other chapters.

Mary Banks and her team at BMJ Publications have ably encouraged and supported us through the book's long gestation and Judith Ockenden copy-edited the manuscript. We also thank Kluwer Academic Publications, Picador Books, Penguin Books, The Lancet, the British Journal of General Practice, the British Medical Journal, the Society for the Social History of Medicine, and the Journal of Medical Ethics for kind permission to reproduce material. Details of these sources and the references of the original works are given at the relevant points in the text.

Professor Marshall Marinker and Professor Howard Brody, whose own work in the field of medical narrative paved the way for this book, gave personal encouragement from the outset. Finally, we owe a special debt to our partners, Fraser Macfarlane and Ruth Richardson, who understood and forgave our preoccupation, and to our children, Robert and Alastair Macfarlane and Joshua Richardson.

Trisha Greenhalgh
Brian Hurwitz
September 1998

Introduction

1 Why study narrative?

Trisha Greenhalgh and Brian Hurwitz

What is narrative?

> One day when Pooh Bear had nothing else to do, he thought he would do something, so he went round to Piglet's house to see what Piglet was doing. It was snowing as he stumped over the white forest track, and he expected to find Piglet warming his toes in front of the fire, but to his surprise he saw that the door was open, and the more he looked inside the more Piglet wasn't there.

This short excerpt from the opening chapter of one of the best-loved children's stories of all time[1] illustrates a number of features of the narrative as a linguistic form. First, it has a finite and longitudinal time sequence – that is, it has a beginning, a series of unfolding events, and (we anticipate) an ending. Second, it presupposes both a narrator and a listener, whose different viewpoints are brought to bear on how the story is told. The same sequence of events, told by another person to another audience, might be presented quite differently without being any less "true".

Third, the narrative is concerned with individuals. Furthermore, it concerns how those individuals *feel* and how people feel about them, rather than simply what they do or what is done to them. Both Pooh Bear, trudging hopefully through the snow, and Piglet, mysteriously absent from his usual place beside the fire, are already *characters* in the story rather than merely the objects of the tale. Fourth, the narrative provides items of information that do not pertain simply or directly to the unfolding of events. This is an important point. In contrast, say, with a list of measurements or a description of the outcome of an experiment, there is no self-evident definition of what is relevant or what is irrelevant in a particular narrative. The choice of what to tell, and what to omit, lies entirely with the narrator (modified, at his or her discretion, by the inquisitive questions of the listener).

Finally, and perhaps most crucially for the purposes of this book, the narrative is absorbing. It engages the listener and invites an

3

interpretation. When you read the example above, you may have fleetingly considered whether Pooh will go out to look for Piglet, or settle down beside the fire to await his return. You may be right, or wrong, if you assume that Pooh is anxious about his friend's safety. If you were to hear more of the story, your original interpretation of the material and emotional situation of Pooh and Piglet might very well change. In short, what the extract offers us is an experience of *"living through,* not simply *knowledge about"* the characters in the story.[2]

If he were allowed to tell his own story, Pooh Bear's *autobiographical* narrative would be a very different account from the one told in the third person. The particular encounters and memories he might choose to disclose may not be those AA Milne has put on record. Life's experiences understood as enacted narrative, as a unique and personal story "put into practice", is a central focus of the insight narrative analysis can offer medical practitioners.

Narratives of clinical interest tend toward plot in their structure rather than the more basic narrative of a simple story. In his book *Aspects of the Novel*, E M Forster explains the difference between these two genres: "in a story we say 'and then – and then' … in a plot we say 'why?'" To the extent that diagnosis involves assimilating diverse aspects of a patient's story with clinical, laboratory and other findings in order to arrive upon a plausible answer to the medical question "why?" (what best explains this particular patient's concatenation of experiences), the question of causality overshadows the patient narrative. "The king died then the queen died" is a story; but "the king died then the queen died of grief" is plot, Forster tells us, because it reveals a deeper meaning within the sequence of events which helps us to understand why the events happened as they did.[3]

As Anna Donald argues cogently in Chapter 2, life has no meaning that exists independently of the stories told about it. This is, of course, literally true in the sense that only that which is narrated can be said to have any meaning. But it is also true in the sense that narration is the forward movement of description of actions and events making possible the backward action of self reflection and self understanding.[4]

You could make an objective list of the actions you performed over the last week, but if it were simply a "factual" account, it would not *mean* anything. But if you *told* us what you had done in the last week, not only would your story acquire meaning, but in telling it, both you the narrator and we the listeners would be compelled to reflect on it in order to gain a greater understanding of what had gone on. We would almost certainly start off the reflecting process using the notions that you had used to make sense of last week's actions. Having yourself told, reflected, and been understood, you may be able to resolve any misgivings about particular events, and perhaps plan future actions. Just as history does not exist in nature, but is created in the telling, so, too autobiography and the medical case history emerge out of transactions which mean they are at the same time both less and more than the 'facts' of the case. Forster believed narrative could be "truer than history because it goes beyond the evidence, and each of us knows from his own experience that there is something beyond the evidence".[3]

Narrative in the experience of illness and healing

Hardy writes that we "dream in narrative, daydream in narrative, remember, anticipate, hope, despair, believe, doubt, plan, revise, criticise, construct, gossip, learn, hate and love by narrative".[5] The clinical experience of health professionals (perhaps particularly in primary care, as Iona Heath argues in Chapter 9) demonstrates that episodes of sickness are, if nothing else, important milestones in the enacted narratives of patients' lives. Thus, not only do we live by narrative, but, often with our doctors and nurses as witnesses,[6] we fall ill, get better, get worse, stay the same and finally die by narrative too.

Similar perceptions underpin John Berger's claim that doctors, in their efforts to intervene and play a role in the unfolding of such stories, become honorary members of innumerable families. The special intimacy that results allows us to enter into people's lives in a unique and privileged way, but free of many of the ties and impediments of real family members. Nevertheless, the health professional's fusion with, and separation from, the narrative streams of very many people – "the dialectic of distance and intimacy"[4] in doctor–patient relationships – cannot exactly replicate that within a family. Such similitude would make the practice of medicine too stressful. Doctors' inability to recall many of the deceased patients they once cared for indicates the limitations of familial relations as the model for doctor–patient relationships. As Brian Hurwitz describes in *Dead notes* (p. 159), family members only rarely forget deceased kin.

Even in the least enlightened backwaters of autocratic and doctor-centred medicine, the patient has always retained a sovereign position as a bearer of information, and the most pompous of professors have been known to chide their students with the warning, "Listen to the patient; s/he's telling you the diagnosis." A more sophisticated view holds that when doctors take a medical history we inevitably act as ethnographers, historians, and biographers, requiring to understand aspects of personhood, personality, social and psychological functioning, as well as biological and physical phenomena.[7]

Thus, patients' narratives provide us with far more than factual information of the kind that might be more efficiently obtained when they are obliged to carry electronic smart cards encoded with their entire "medical history". Indeed, several authors in this book (see in particular Chapters 10, 11, 18, and 24) suggest that the holy grail of "pure" factual information in the clinical encounter is a spurious quest, and in Chapter 19 Steve Kay and Ian Purves argue forcefully for a facility for recording the "story stuff" in the computerised medical record.

The narrative provides meaning, context, and perspective for the patient's predicament. It defines how, why, and in what way he or she is ill. It offers, in short, a possibility of *understanding* which cannot be arrived at by any other means. This is why doctors and therapists alike frequently see their role in terms of facilitating "alternative stories that make sense from the patient's point of view."[8][9] Indeed, Jeremy Holmes (in Chapter 18) goes further and suggests that the role of the therapist is to assist the patient in his or her attempt to construct and work through the *unconscious* elements of a half-written personal story.

Writing on the relationships between language, thought and reality, Benjamin Whorf discussed how

> ... we dissect nature along lines laid down by our native languages. The categories and types that we isolate from the world of phenomena we do not find there because they stare every observer in the face; on the contrary ... the world is organised by our minds – and this means largely by the linguistic systems in our minds. We cut up, organise it into concepts, and ascribe significances ... .[10]

As the examples in Boxes 1.2 and 1.3 show, and as summarised in Box 1.1, understanding the narrative context of illness provides a framework for approaching a patient's problems holistically, as well as revealing potential diagnostic and therapeutic options which we ignore at the patient's peril. Furthermore, illness narratives provide a medium for education of patient and professional, and expand and enrich the research agenda. As Kathryn Montgomery Hunter describes in the evocatively named article "Don't think zebras",[11] medical students rely crucially on anecdotes of extreme and atypical cases in order to develop the essential ability to question expectations, interrupt stereotyped thought patterns, and adjust to new developments as a case unfolds.

The dialogue in Box 1.2 took place between one of us and a patient attending a diabetic clinic in general practice. The patient, originally from Glasgow, now lives in London. The conversation was recorded on tape and is reproduced almost verbatim with the patient's consent. There are a number of important points in the story. First, the immediacy of the patient's voice, his particular way of explaining things, cannot be ignored by a listener or reader, though this would be impossible to capture were the story to be retold in the standard medical history form. Second, the onset of this man's disease is inextricably embedded in a narrative structure: he

---

Box 1.1: Why study narratives?

In the *diagnostic encounter*, narratives:

- are the phenomenal form in which patients experience ill health;
- encourage empathy and promote understanding between clinician and patient;
- allow construction of meaning;
- may supply useful analytical clues and categories.

In the *therapeutic process*, narratives:

- encourage a holistic approach to management;
- are themselves intrinsically therapeutic or palliative;
- may suggest or precipitate additional therapeutic options.

In the *education* of patients and professionals, narratives:

- are often memorable;
- are grounded in experience;
- enforce reflection.

In *research*, narratives:

- set a patient-centred agenda;
- challenge received wisdom;
- generate new hypotheses.

Box 1.2: Robert's story

BH How long have you been diabetic for?

RG Since September 1969.

BH Tell me how you first found out that you were diabetic.

RG Well my tongue started to get very, very dry and also I was drinking excessive amounts of liquid and also I had an upset stomach. So I went to my doctor and told him all this, and all he told me was that I had an "upset stomach" and I told him then that I think I am a diabetic and he told me that I was talking a load of rubbish.

BH Why did your symptoms suggest diabetes to you?

RG Because I have been with a diabetic before who has now died. I had known him since he was 9 years old, so the symptoms I had he described to me before and that is how I knew I thought I was a diabetic. So I went to another doctor and he told me the same thing, that I had an upset stomach. So I waited and waited and waited, then I decided to go back to my doctor, when my water was starting to crystallise and he told me that I had VD.

BH What do you mean by "when my water started to crystallise"? How did you know your water was crystallising?

RG When I was passing the water the end of my penis started getting all white and also some times when the water hit the pan it was starting to go clear white.

BH What happened next?

RG Well, I decided to go down to the VD clinic down in London and I went in there on the Friday night and I handed him the letter and he read it and he said to me "what do you think you have got" and I said "I think I have got diabetes" and he said "what F-ing B sent you here, he should have seen this before you were sent here". So he said to me "look I cannot do anything for you tonight, but please report down to the hospital the next morning (and that was Saturday morning)". So I went back home and I came down the Saturday morning, but with me walking down on the Friday night and the Saturday morning which normally takes me about 5 minutes, took me 35 minutes just to reach the bus stop.

BH Why was that?

RG Because I was so weak I could hardly move at all. So I went down, got down to hospital, went in and told the Sister and the receptionist that I would like to see somebody from the Diabetic Clinic and she read the letter then she told me that I could not get an appointment until a fortnight. At this stage I was really very angry and I started shouting at her. As that started a nurse came out from Casualty and she read the letter. As soon as she read the letter she shouted to a nurse to get a wheelchair, she dumped me in the wheelchair and took me straight upstairs to the Diabetic Clinic. So once I got up there they stripped me off right down to my underpants and started testing me. There was 2 doctors and 3 nurses there and after they stripped me and everything they transferred me over to the hospital. Since the nurse read the letter and took me over to hospital it only took 22 minutes.

BH When you arrived on the ward at the hospital did the doctors tell you what level your blood sugar was at?

RG No they did not. They only told me it was very, very high and a nurse came over with a jug which held 2 gallons of water and she told me that I had to drink that as fast as I could.

BH = Dr Brian Hurwitz

RG = Patient

recounts the symptoms as they unfolded with almost choreographic precision together with his efforts to communicate them.

Despite the passage of 30 years, the patient's utter helplessness at the hands of his personal medical attendants is chilling. It is not simply that his doctor did not appear to listen to him; the doctor's advice and inaction were predicated upon an entirely different story from the one that required urgent intervention. Richard Asher was graphic in drawing our attention to the dangerous tendency of clinicians to see the expected and unconsciously to dismiss the anomalous: "we have to beware of this suppressive faculty which, by producing selective deafness, selective blindness and other sense rejections, can so easily suppress the significant and the relevant."[12]

In RG's case, the medical focus had apparently centred upon the bowel disturbance and appeared to discount the patient's personal knowledge of diabetes and his evident ability to make sense of a set of diverse symptoms. The acuteness of the patient's own observations was pertinent. Indeed, if specks of white glucose upon patent leather shoes deserve a photograph in a textbook of diabetic physical signs,[13] then the white jet stream forming when glucose-loaded urine crystallises in the lavatory pan should make the astute clinician sit up and take notice.

The authenticity, uniqueness, and deep contextual meaning of the illness narrative told in the first person, clearly demonstrated in the example in Box 1.2, comes across strongly in the personal accounts of illness by Stephen Jay Gould, Robert McCrum and Donald Bateman, reproduced in Chapters 3, 4, and 5 respectively, and in the anonymous accounts in Gillie Bolton's *Stories of dying* (Chapter 6) and Henrietta Weinbren and Paramjit Gill's *Have I got epilepsy or has it got me?* (Chapter 7). All these accounts are to a large extent "anecdotal" – that is, they reflect the personal experience of the narrator rather than the aggregated experiences of a population sample. Jane Macnaughton reminds us (Chapter 20) that anecdote brings a number of advantages as well as the well documented problem of "bias". Among other things, anecdotes or "illness scripts" are the form in which we accumulate our medical or nursing knowledge.[14 15]

The case in Box 1.3 shows how biographical forces can be mobilised therapeutically. The strategy that successfully helped the patient stop smoking pressed into service a central value held by the patient – the importance, to a lawyer, of keeping to one's side of a contract. More attuned to the latent opportunities of

---

Box 1.3: A treatment plan with meaning

A man in his mid forties had consulted me on many occasions over the previous 3 years saying he wanted to give up smoking. I tried several approaches including advice, trying to mobilise his will power by focusing upon his feelings of stigma, especially in respect and his children's fierce opposition to the habit. Leaflets, and nicotine replacement therapy, were no help – he did not manage to quit for more than a week. He eventually referred himself to a complementary practitioner who advised him to draw up a legal contract with himself. This was to state the date on which he intended to quit, and was to be signed and witnessed. From that due date he never smoked again.

---

intervening in a patient's story, the alternative practitioner succeeded in harnessing the narrative elements to hand, where the conventional doctor (one of us) had failed, despite the growing evidence-base on the effectiveness of conventional smoking cessation interventions.

The study of meaning

The notion of interpretation (the discernment of meaning) is a central concern of philosophers and linguists, but it is a concept with which doctors and other scientists are often unfamiliar, and hence uncomfortable. We recognise, but we cannot elucidate with our familiar scientific tools, the meaning that narrative gives to sequences of events, a meaning that usually binds agents and events within intelligible patterns, and which asserts a particular human significance, whether symbolic, biographical or biological.[4] To make progress with understanding meaning, we must look to literature rather than science. Stephen Rachman (Chapter 13) suggests some classic texts to start with, and Harriet Squier (Chapter 14) suggests *how* modules on literature and the humanities can be used to augment a traditional medical school curriculum. In addition, at the end of the book, we have included an appendix of recommended reading.

Hunter, a professor of literature with a strong involvement in medical education, writes that clinical medicine "shares its methods of knowing with history, law, economics, anthropology, and other human sciences less certain and more concerned with meaning than the physical sciences. But unlike those disciplines, it does not explicitly recognise its interpretive character or the rules it uses to negotiate meaning."[11] She admits to being puzzled by the medical profession's preoccupation with the gold standard of science in clinical practice, and believes that medicine is better characterised as a "moral knowing, a narrative, interpretive, practical reasoning,"[16 17] an argument which we cover in more depth in Chapter 24.

At its most arid, modern medicine lacks a metric for existential qualities such as inner hurt, despair, hope, grief, and moral pain which frequently accompany, and often indeed constitute, the illnesses from which people suffer.[18] Quality of life measures reflect one approach to such a metric, but almost always involve reduction of quality into quantity and the imposition of the values and preferences of one person or group on others.[19] Marshall Marinker's description of Hilda Thomson (Chapter 11) illustrates this point. The complexity and "beingness" of the patient depicted by Marinker underpin the calls made in the USA to substitute "chief complaint" and "complains of" sections of the typical case history with an "existential complaint" formulation, that can convey knowledge about the personal world and suffering of the patient.

Weinbren's qualitative research study of children telling and drawing the stories of their illness (Chapter 7) offers a sobering insight into what it *means* to live a life blighted by epilepsy. The quotations from Weinbren's study demonstrate that narratives, in expressing our own attempts to make sense of our lives, usually presuppose causation. Indeed, the philosopher William James believed that our very notion of causality is "...but an empty name covering simply a demand that the sequence of events shall one day manifest a deeper kind of belonging of one thing with another than the mere arbitrary juxtaposition which now phenomenally appears".[20] Since patients almost invariably place their most important experiences – birth, death, grief, and illness – within very different narrative streams than do doctors, it follows that doctors and patients often assign very different meanings (and different streams of causality) to the same sequence of events.

The transactional way in which facts emerge in the doctor–patient relationship indicates that as well as being potential readers of such texts, health professionals need to understand their role in authoring "the text-that-is-the-patient". It should therefore not surprise us that the sorts of concerns we have when reading literature – whose voice is the narrator's, where does the chain of causation begin, whom can we believe? – arise constantly in conversations between patients and health professionals.[16] In Chapter 10, John Launer argues that the tension between the complex narrative which the patient brings into the consulting room and the doctor's account of what is *really* going on is particularly acute in psychiatry, a field which he describes as "an uncomfortable no-man's land between conventional medical science and a search for meaning which extends into political and religious domains", but also as "the only area of specialist medicine where talking and listening are explicitly understood to be therapeutic."

The multiplicity of readings which a text engenders is precisely what makes the narrative such an absorbing form, and the implications of this are explored further by Anne Hudson Jones in *Narrative in medical ethics* (Chapter 21) and Brian Hurwitz in *The wounded storyteller* (Chapter 23). In *Nursing, narrative and the moral imagination* (Chapter 16), P. Anne Scott suggests that it is by becoming finely aware of the various possible "readings" of the patient's unfinished story that we appreciate fully the moral choices in health care.

A lost tradition

In some ways, the narratives we read in books, whose form is already set on the printed page, are less interesting than those we hear in what is called the "oral tradition".[21] The stories of myths and legends, continually re-created by word of mouth in successive generations, still feature prominently in many non-Western societies and impact profoundly on the experience of health and illness[22] (a theme which is taken up by Vieda Skultans in Chapter 22).

It is perhaps because Western culture has lost its grip on the oral tradition that the skills of listening to, appreciating, and interpreting patients' stories are only rarely upheld as core clinical skills in the medical curriculum.[23] Indeed, much of the current emphasis in medical training is on the student acquiring the ability to express a patient's problem in the structured and standardised format that has come to be known as the "medical history" in the UK and the "clinical clerking" in the USA.[23] It has been shown that, somewhere between the first year and the final year of medical education, undergraduate students *exchange* a native facility for eliciting and appreciating patients' narratives for the learned expertise of constructing a medical history.[24]

Over the past 200 years or so, the patient's narrative has become increasingly repressed in medical practice, as Stuart Hogarth and Lara Marks explain in Chapter 15. But as Sir Richard Bayliss recounts in Chapter 8, narrative frequently appears in a vestigial form even in the conventional clinical encounter of modern times. Certain symptom descriptions, for example, appear as fragments torn from elaborate stories and alighted upon by clinicians as especially revelatory: "My shortness of breath always gets worse when I lie down but the funny thing is the pain only comes on when I climb stairs"; or, "I was washing the dishes when everything went black – it was like a curtain coming down". Less familiar experiences may be just as important to the patient, but the value of such classical symptoms to physicians as readers of signs is akin to a mirror held up to nature: the story fragments faithfully portray, in a linguistic form, particular biological dysfunctions, so closely are they aligned to physiological and pathological mechanisms.

The relentless substitution during the course of medical training of skills that are fundamentally linguistic, empathic and inter-pretive for those deemed "scientific", eminently measurable but unavoidably reductionist, should be seen as anything but a successful feature of the modern curriculum. Over 30 years ago, the then President of the Royal College of Physicians lamented that "The first staggering fact about medical education is that after two and a half years of being taught on the assumption that everyone is the same the student has to find out for himself that everyone is different, which is what his experience has taught him since infancy",[25] a sentiment echoed more recently by J Campbell Murdoch in his lecture *Mackenzie's puzzle – the cornerstone of teaching and research in general practice.*[26]

The conventional clinical case history – the standardised features of the illness experience which doctors and medical students select from the patient's narrative – represents, at best, the intersection between a particular patient world and the abstract world of medical knowledge, about which patients may know little. The core clinical skills of listening, questioning, delineating, marshalling, explaining and interpreting provide a potential mediation between

13

these different worlds. Yet as Michael Balint pointed out, whether these tasks are performed well or badly is likely to have as much influence on the outcome of the illness from the patient's point of view as the more scientific and technical aspects of diagnosis or treatment.[27][28]

It was as a result of prolonged and protected discussions with general practitioners caught within, and troubled by, long-term patient relationships that Michael Balint recognised the importance of narrative entanglement in clinical work. Prior to Balint's work in the 1950s, the clinical story had been dominated by one particular narrative genre. Arising towards the end of 18th century from very different doctor–patient relationships to those of Balint's discussants (see Chapter 15), the clinical case history began to depict patient stories in solely medico-technical terms.[29] Often dominated by considerations of diagnosis or the "natural history" of disease progression as revealed by changing symptoms and signs, or by the results of particular clinical manoeuvres and laboratory tests, the clinical case history became a refracted depersonalised account unrecognisable to the patient, whose legacy we recognise today. With its focus upon correlating clinico-pathological findings, it has been enormously influential both in forwarding medical understanding of complex clinical phenomena, and in regulating doctor–patient relationships.

It is surely no accident that Marshall Marinker, who drew such perceptive lessons from the story of Hilda Thomson in the 1970s (reproduced here in Chapter 11), was a member of one of Balint's original study groups. The Balint groups attended by general practitioners in the 1950s and 60s, and the ongoing tradition of this approach, did much to sustain and disseminate his teaching on the value of narrative in the consultation and continuing care. This legacy probably had considerable influence on how medicine is taught, particularly to general practitioners in training. But it has not, for the most part, led to measurable changes in the way medicine is practised or accredited, and it has not given rise to a significant programme of systematic research into the analysis and therapeutic use of narrative in the consultation.

In *Stories we hear and stories we tell* (Chapter 17), Glyn Jones Elwyn and Richard Gwyn provide us with a taste of the emerging discipline of narrative analysis in the context of health care, and remind us how partial our current understanding is of what our patients are saying to us. We hope that this book will go some way towards redressing that deficit.

1 Milne AA. *The house at Pooh corner.* London: Methuen & Co, 1974 (first published 1928).
2 Rosenblatt LM. Literature as exploration. NewYork: MLA, 1983. Quoted in Anderson C. Literature and medicine: why should the physician read ... or write? In: Peterfreund S. ed. *Literature and science.* Boston, USA: Northeastern University Press, 1990.
3 Forster E M. *Aspects of the novel.* Harmondsworth, Middlesex: Penguin Books, 1971, p. 70.
4 Churchill LR, Churchill SW. Storytelling in medical arenas: the art of self-determination. *Lit Med* 1982; **1**: 73–9.
5 Hardy B. Towards a poetics of fiction: an approach through narrative. *Novel* 1986; 5–14. Quoted in: Widdershoven G. The story of life: hermeneutic perspectives on the relationship between narrative and life history. In Josselson R, Lieblich A eds *The narrative study of lives.* London: Sage Publications, 1993.
6 Berger J, Mohr J. *A fortunate man: the story of a country doctor.* Harmondsworth, Middlesex: Penguin Books, 1967.
7 Epstein J. *Altered conditions: disease, medicine and storytelling.* New York and London: Routledge, 1995.
8 Launer J, Lindsey C. Training for systemic general practice: a new approach from the Tavistock Clinic. *Br J Gen Pract* 1997; **47**: 453–6.
9 Brody H. My story is broken; can you help me fix it? *Lit Med* 1994; **13**: 79–92.
10 Benjamin Lee Whorf. Science and linguistics. In: Carroll JB. ed. *Language, thought, and reality: selected writings of Benjamin Lee Whorf.* Quoted in Peterfreund S ed. *Literature and science.* Boston, USA: Northeastern University Press, 1990.
11 Hunter K. "Don't think zebras": uncertainty, interpretation, and the place of paradox in clinical education. *Theoret Med* 1996; **17**: 225–41.
12 Asher R. *Clinical sense.* The 1959 Lettsomian Lectures. In: Avery Jones F ed. *Richard Asher talking sense.* London: Pitman Books Ltd, 1972, p. 3.
13 Bloom A and Ireland R? *A colour atlas of diabetes.* London: Wolfe Medical Publications, 1980, p. 17.
14 Schmidt HG, Norman GR, Boshuizen HPA. A cognitive perspective on medical expertise: theory and implications. *Academ Med* 1990; **65**: 611–21.
15 Custers EJ, Boshuizen HP, Schmidt HG. The influence of medical expertise, case typicality, and illness script component on case processing and disease probability estimates. *Mem Cognit* 1996; **24**: 384–99.
16 Hunter KM. Narrative, literature, and the clinical exercise of practical reason. *J Med Phil* 1996; **21**: 303–20.
17 Hunter KM. *Doctors' stories.* Princeton, USA: Princeton University Press, 1991, p. 12.
18 Kleinman A. *The illness narratives.* NewYork, USA: Basic Books, 1988.
19 Hopkins A. *Measures of the quality of life and the uses to which such measures may be put.* London: Royal College of Physicians, 1992.
20 James W. The dilemma of determinism. In: James W. *TheWill to Believe and Other Essays in Popular Philosophy.* NewYork: Dover, 1956 (first published 1897).
21 Ratzan RM. Winged words and chief complaints: medical case histories and the Parry-Lord oral-formulaic tradition. *Lit Med* 1992; **11**: 94–114.
22 Helman C. *Culture, Health and Illness*, 3rd edition. London: Butterworth Heinemann, 1994.
23 Lowry S. *Learning Medicine.* London: BMJ Publications, 1995.
24 Preven DW, Kachur EK, Kupfer RB, Walters JA. Interviewing skills of first year medical students. *J Med Educat* 1986; **61**: 842–4.
25 Platt R. Thoughts on teaching medicine. *Br Med J* 1965; **2**: 551–2.
26 Murdoch JC. Mackenzie's puzzle – the cornerstone of teaching and research in general practice. *Br J Gen Pract* 1997; **47**: 656–8.
27 Balint E and Norrell J eds. *Six minutes for the patient: interactions in general practice consultations.* London: Tavistock Publications, 1973.

28 Balint M. *The doctor, his patient and the illness.* London: Tavistock Publications, 1957.
29 Fissell ME. The disappearance of the patient's narrative and the invention of hospital medicine. In: French R, Wear A eds. *British medicine in an age of reform.* London and New York: Routledge, 1991, pp. 92–109.

2   The words we live in

Anna Donald

As other pieces in this book describe, people experience illness within a narrative, or story, that shapes and gives meaning to what they are feeling, moment to moment. The story of Robert's diabetes (page 8) is a powerful account of both the physical symptoms and the variety of emotions that accompanied the delayed diagnosis and inappropriate treatment of a life-threatening illness. The description by Harriet's father in Chapter 7 shows how the experience of epilepsy by both the child and the family changed as the various specialist opinions were sought, provisional diagnoses offered, treatments tried, and investigations endured.

Illness narratives are noticeable because they are usually different from those of the rest of our lives. But narratives are not unique to illness, nor to patients. Over the past 40 years, the social sciences have been transformed by the understanding that human beings live within and embody socially constructed narratives from which they cannot be extricated; that you or I would be essentially different people were we to have been raised in a different culture or at a different time. Clifford Geertz, one of the early authors of this world view, explained this in 1961:[1]

> More bluntly, [this theory] suggests that there is no such thing as a human nature independent of culture ... . As our central nervous system – and most particularly its crowning curse and glory, the neocortex – grew up in great part in interaction with culture, it is incapable of directing our behavior or organizing our experience without the guidance provided by systems of significant symbols ... . Such symbols are thus not mere expressions, instrumentalities, or correlates of our biological, psychological, and social existence; they are prerequisites of it. Without men, no culture, certainly; but equally, and more significantly, without culture, no men.

With notable exceptions,[2] these insights into how humans work have yet to percolate directly into most health professionals' training or practice. In this largely derivative piece, therefore, I aim to describe and speculate a little further on the process by which we construct narratives within which we live, and how common differences in health-related narratives – for example, between patients and doctors, or between homeopaths and allopathic practitioners – can seem like conflicts between what is *real*, rather than struggles for whose narrative becomes the dominant one.

Many philosophers and anthropologists have pointed out that as human beings, we live within narratives, or stories, of which we are the principle authors.[3] Only, just as we do not consciously perceive how our retina processes light signals, but only the optical images that result, we are unconscious of the way in which we create our own narratives, seeing only the images produced that we mistakenly perceive as *real*: blue sky; shiny car; rich woman; tired Peter. While physics suggests that the sky, car, woman, and Peter are nothing more than empty spaces containing more or less probable electrons, our story-telling capacity enables us to make something of this sub-atomic chaos, imposing order and predictability onto it and allowing us to make meaningful contact with other people across the void. It also allows us to be creative: to invent new stories to live by, and therefore to create new realities for ourselves, even though we remain largely unconscious of our own creative acts. For example, the narrative describing how diseases such as cholera were caused by miasmas was eventually replaced in the 19th century by the narrative of invading microbes, which proved to be a more effective means of organising new notions of disease and hygiene. The microbial narrative still holds sway, but with the recent discovery of prions and further investigations into the genetic components of viruses, it is at least plausible that we may be in for a new kind of infectious disease narrative within the next 50 years.

How do we create narratives, individually and collectively? At present, linguists and psychologists think that, unlike other mammals, we seem to be born with the capacity for symbolisation – in language and other forms of self expression – and for narrative structure, including the ability to generate grammar.[4] In virtually all cultures it does seem that from the moment humans are born, they become story-telling machines, struggling to acquire new words, or more broadly, new symbols, and new ways of putting them together. We learn from older human beings, including our parents, words with which to spin our stories as well as narrative structures in which to place them, even though we are rarely conscious of this process of symbol and narrative-attainment: Dad; ball; apple juice. To some extent, this learning process continues all our lives as we come into contact with new words, new ways of putting them together, and new sensations to express: as teenagers finding ways to say emerging feelings of sexuality and responsibility; as parents finding ways of talking to offspring; as elders finding ways of speaking to death. As patients, we find ways to express lost freedoms;[5] as medical students, to express the visual array of human tissue and bodily mechanisms; a way of seeing that Foucault called "the Gaze".

I would add further that the symbolic/story-making process is not an abstract one that goes on somewhere in the intellect, or solely in the white and grey matter of the cortex. Rather, that in relay with the brain, narratives are processed and programmed into the rest of the body: the musculature and autonomic nervous system; that whole domain of feelings: of rage, of pain, of joy, the felt responses to information that we carelessly call emotions. It certainly feels as if my muscles and joints, as well as my neurones, respond to narratives: "Granny has died". But I would add also that the supposedly dumb body is integrally involved not just in responding, but in the creation and embedding of narratives, and that this involvement is what transforms idle musing into supposed reality, when "normative categories" become "descriptive terms". That sticks and stones may break my bones but names can never hurt me – that is, until I embed those names in the musculature of my body; and in so doing, make them real. Then they become bullets, not merely the taunts of the ignorant, and can hurt me very much. And that this linkage of symbols to bodily feelings is perhaps one of the main reasons that narratives have such power in directing our actions, as well as being so difficult to change. For if my world view is literally wired up to my autonomic nervous system rather than being an abstract constellation of feeling-less thoughts, then it is likely to take more than a rational debate to alter it.

Many have described the conservative tendency of narrative structures.[7-9] For example, it usually takes a new generation before immigrant families "assimilate" to their new surroundings. Perhaps this is because it is literally too difficult for the first-generation migrants to disconnect physically from narratives of the old country and re-connect themselves to those of the society they now find themselves in, whereas for their children it is not so hard, although the new generation faces a different task of reconciling the narratives of their parents with those of the new country. Similarly, each generation finds new ways of distinguishing itself from the last by creating and embedding in their bodies new narratives. Teenage rebellion at least partly involves the creation – and somatisation – of new narratives that distinguish the child from the parent, and which are therefore almost by definition likely to cause conflict over whose version of reality is the right one. Parents use all kinds of methods to try to prevent their children from making the new narratives real (that is, from somatising them), through which they might lose them into a different narrative – and hence, literally, a different reality.

Yet, while made conservative perhaps through somatisation, narratives are ultimately human creations, and as such *are* changeable – and do change. Like genes, narratives change over time and distance, and can sometimes be traced to common ancestors, encapsulated in myths and legends. Doctors' lives are riddled with practices that have evolved from earlier narratives about what constituted sensible behaviour, such as routinely collecting blood from patients (bleeding the body of impurities), thinning the blood with anticoagulants (to cool the body down), and giving out pills (in a ritual of gift-giving), even when we know them to be useless, such as antibiotics for viral illnesses.[10]

Why do we create narratives with such facility, and so unconsciously? One possible explanation is an evolutionary one: without our story-making process, it would be difficult to survive, because narratives give us the capacity to navigate and to order our senses and thereby the world. Young babies see their parents as blobs and splotches, not because their retinas are undeveloped, but because they lack any kind of narrative distinction of Mum or Dad with which to organise the myriad sensations (smell, sight, hearing, touch, feelings) exciting their cells. Perceiving only blobs and splotches may not pose a threat to survival while parents keep vigil nearby, but the infant would not last long were she to be left to her own devices in such a random universe. Just as baby deer learn quickly to run for survival, human babies learn quickly to distinguish, and later to say, words and phrases for the constellations of senses that accompany Mum, Dad, milk, bath. In doing so, they gradually become less dependent upon their parents, and less likely to succumb to an undistinguished danger.

Narrative construction is not, however, confined to babies, but rather is a lifelong process that enables adults also to navigate new experiences, as they also encounter new things they do not always have ready-made distinctions for. Take wine, for example. The wine buff will ooh and aah over the hints of vanilla, the whiffs of citrus, the edge of mineral in what to the rest of us tastes like, well, white wine. But a few evenings in wine class, where we learn some wine distinctions and how to put them into wine narratives – to describe one smell/taste/colour sensation as cinnamon, and another as eucalyptus, and that the oaks of Australian chardonnays are often too heavy – and we'll be oohing and aahing with the best of them.

Without intelligible narratives, we are lost. For example, it would seem that until we begin to develop language, we have difficulty in forming conscious memories, as we have no narrative structure within which to formulate it. The blind and deaf girl, Helen Keller, reported that she only began to remember her life from the age of five, when she distinguished her first word, *water*, from the sensation of water running on to her hand at the same time as her teacher signed the word into her other palm.[11] Children, such as orphans in neglectful institutions, who for lack of adult contact do not learn the process of creating their own narratives, cannot function as social beings until someone teaches them how.[12] And when people's narratives for navigating the world and symbolising feelings become unintelligible – that is, when their experiences and feelings outstrip their capacity to distinguish and say them – people usually become physically and mentally ill, as they did in droves following the daily insanity of the concentration camps of World War II,[13] or the senseless guerrilla warfare of Vietnam, following which more men died from suicide than were killed in action.

Narratives bind us socially with others; without shared narratives, we become socially isolated and also ill. Solitary confinement has long been used as a form of extreme punishment, while self-help organisations such as Alcoholics Anonymous strive to create a narrative structure in which people isolated in their stories, and further isolated by drink, can join together in a shared narrative and subsequently recover from their suffering. Numerous studies have demonstrated that people's rates of illness and accidents rise dramatically following profound losses, such as bereavement, divorce, and other losses of people or things that support narrative structures, and that thereby isolate the individual from his social, or interpretive community.[14 15] For example, death of children, which opposes most cultures' narratives about what children represent – life, the future, reproduction, fertility, hope – causes, on average, much more severe suffering, and greater illness prevalence for those left behind than the death of old people, for which we are amply endowed with stories to explain their passing.

Problems arise when people assume (as we all do) that their

individual and community's distinctions and narratives *are reality* – for them and for everyone else – rather than just a set of arbitrary (although conservative) metaphors for organising and making predictable infinite permutations and combinations of sensations. That Jesus rather than Mohammed saved the world; that herpes is a virus, that women are smarter than men. As Clifford Geertz pointed out in the 1960s, wars are fought not over what the truth is, but over people's struggle for the right to assert their version of it.[16]

Such conflicts are common in health care settings, in which different social groups frequently hold different distinctions and explanatory frameworks, or narratives, for identifying and navigating illness, as pieces in this book testify. For example, the main cause of a bout of influenza and its best means of management will vary greatly depending on whether you consult with a chest physician, a psychotherapist, a yoga guru, an acupuncturist, a homeopath, a public health doctor, or someone actually suffering from its severest symptoms, such as pain and high fever. As Susan Sontag pointed out long ago, the perceived causes and appropriate treatment of many diseases, from tuberculosis and cancer to AIDS,[17 18] have varied widely over time and between social groups, according to meta-narratives of disease as punishment, as purification, as a sign of holiness, virtue, idleness or poverty; as the result of imbalances in the body or of invading organisms. Of course, it is perfectly normal to hold several of these explanatory narratives concurrently. Most people bargain with God when seriously ill,[19] promising to be more virtuous in the future, while simultaneously taking medicines to address the cause of the illness as defined by the microbe narrative of Western medicine.

What constitutes a particular disease (such as influenza) is also frequently contested, noticeably between those working in different cultural systems. For example, traditional Chinese medicine, with its different explanatory narratives for physiology of the body and causes of illness, identifies many diseases that Western medicine does not, while omitting others, such as depression, that cannot be easily explained within its energy-based aetiological framework, nor which are socially acceptable, even in modern-day China.[20]

Within Western medicine itself there continues to arise new and conflicting narratives of disease identity, causation and treatment. Each, for a time, rocks the scientific boat as different factions take sides as to whether the newcomer is worthy of "reality" status (a marker of which is its being included within the directory of successful medical metaphors, the *International Classification of Diseases*), or whether it should be relegated to the scrap-heap of misguided hypotheses. Not so long ago, coronary heart disease was contested as a recognisable disease,[21] while battles still rage over conditions such as post traumatic stress disorder,[22] myalgic encephalitis (ME),[23] and bovine spongiform encephalopathy (BSE) in humans. Arguably much of the function of medical research is to provide evidence for or against metaphorical systems and thereby to help establish narratives secure enough for people to navigate their illness experience by. Secure narratives are not necessarily those that include cure or even symptom relief (many recognised neurological conditions exclude both), but are those in which the sufferer's symptoms are recognised as *socially* legitimate and which enable the sufferer to be included within his interpretive communities. As Arthur Kleinman vividly describes in his case-studies of patients suffering from chronic pain but lacking medical diagnoses, woe betide the patient whose symptoms are not recognised by the ICD classification system, and who thereby risks becoming a social pariah of the worst kind: malingerer, liar or lunatic.[24]

Conflicts in narratives about illness and disease also arise between health professionals and patients. One type of conflict arises from an ontological mismatch between the sufferer's actual experience of illness and the health professional's reformulation of it as disease. For example, while the patient might *feel* pain, fever and an aching throat, the clinician *sees* viral proliferation of influenza A. Illness is a realm that the ill person *inhabits*, whereas disease categories are often quite crude maps that health professionals use to interpret the ill person's experience, from the other side of the wellness–illness divide. As Susan Sontag described in *Illness as Metaphor*,

> illness is the night-side of life, a more onerous citizenship. Everyone who is born holds dual citizenship, in the kingdom of the well and in the kingdom of the sick. Although we all prefer to use only the good passport, sooner or later each of us is obliged, at least for a spell, to identify ourselves as citizens of that other place.[25]

While, to some extent, differences in narrative are inevitable between the clinician (a well person) and the patient (inhabiting illness), problems arise when clinicians use their disease-category narratives to dominate patients' illness narratives to such an extent that the patients' are obliterated, leaving them demoralised, and sometimes, misdiagnosed. Oliver Sacks' surgeon missed major denervation of Sack's leg when he failed to listen to his patient's doubts about the success of his operation. Sacks describes his demoralization and feelings of despair:

> I was stunned. All the agonized, agonizing uncertainties and fears, all the torment I had suffered since I discovered my condition, all the hopes and expectations I had pinned on this meeting – and now this! I thought: what sort of doctor, what sort of person, is this? He didn't even listen to me ... .[26]

Finally, problems may arise when health professionals hold different narratives from ill people about the identity, cause and therefore best management for their illnesses. For example, it is common in routine medical practice for either the doctor or the patient to attribute the patient's symptoms to psychological distress of various kinds, while the other party attributes it to "physical" disease processes.[27] Similarly, it is common for health professionals and patients from different ethnic groups, or different generations or social classes, to hold different causative frameworks for presenting symptoms.

The recent and rapid development of "evidence based medicine" (EBM) throughout Western medical systems as a statistical method of interrogating fact and fiction in health care is probably most helpful not because it divines some kind of absolute truth, but because it creates a discursive space in which previously conflicting narratives of cause and effect can be reconciled, and warring factions brought to truce. Unlike most other epistemological systems in medicine, EBM does not require faith in any single health narrative. Rather than asking "how does your treatment work?" or "how does your illness feel?" it asks patients and practitioners of all kinds, "did the treatment work, compared with no (or alternative) treatment?" To date, in Britain at least, people from all persuasions are rushing to embrace EBM: from orthopaedic surgeons to homeopaths and expectant mothers. Of course, EBM is hardly narrative-free, itself existing within a modern narrative described by Ian Hacking[28] that upholds relative truth revealed through statistical odds, rather than through priestly oracles or the pronouncement of professional experts. The death of the expert as truth-giver espoused in EBM is reminiscent of the denouncement of priestly experts that took place during the

Reformation. It will be interesting to see over time to what extent it contributes, or disappoints, its early followers.

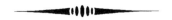

1 Geertz, C. *The Interpretation of Cultures.* New York: Basic Books, 1973 (reprint), p. 49.
2 For example, see Kleinman A. *Rethinking Psychiatry. From Cultural Category to Personal Experience.* New York: The Free Press, 1988; or Desjarlais R, Eisenberg L, Good B, Kleinman A. *World Mental Health. Problems and Priorities in Low-Income Countries.* Oxford: Oxford University Press, 1995.
3 For example, Geertz G. *The Interpretation of Cultures.* New York: Basic Books, 1973; MacIntyre A, The Virtues, the Unity of a Human Life and the Concept of a Tradition. In Sandel M ed. *Liberalism and Its Critics.* Oxford: Blackwell, 1984, pp. 125–48; Fish S. *Doing What Comes Naturally. Change, Rhetoric, and the Practice of Theory in Literary and Legal Studies.* Durham: Duke University Press, 1995; Rorty R. *Contingency, Irony, Solidarity.* Cambridge: Cambridge University Press, 1989.
4 Pinker S. *The Language Instinct. How the Mind Creates Language.* New York: Harperperennial Library, 1995.
5 For a vivid description of the experience of lost freedoms in illness, see Sacks O. *A leg to stand on.* New York: Summit Books, 1984.
6 Foucault M. *Birth of the Clinic. An Archaeology of Medical Perception.* London: Tavistock Publications, 1974.
7 Gadamer HG. *Truth and Method.* New York: Seabury Press, 1975.
8 Fish S. Change. *Doing What Comes Naturally. Rhetoric and the Practice of Theory and Legal Studies.* Durham: Duke University Press, 1989, pp. 141–62.
9 Rorty R. The Contingency of Language. In Goodman RB ed. *Pragmatism: A Contemporary Reader.* New York: Routledge, 1995, pp. 104–24.
10 For one of many good explanations of this process, see Good BJ. Semiotics and the study of medical reality. *Medicine, rationality, and experience. An anthropological perspective.* Cambridge: Cambridge University Press, 1994, pp. 88–115.
11 Keller H. *Story of My Life.* New York: Doubleday, 1991.
12 Hodes, M. Refugee children. *Br Med J* 1998; **316**: 793–4.
13 Felman S, Laub D. *Testimony. Crises of Witnessing in Literature, Psychoanalysis, and History.* New York: Routledge, 1992.
14 Stanley Fish describes the interpretive community as a group of people who share common narratives – and thereby become a coherent social group. See Ref. 3.
15 The British newspaper, *The Independent,* reported during the Bosnian war how one young woman escaped to London, only to find that the lack of people who could share her narratives about the war was so painfully isolating that she preferred to return with her children to war-torn Sarajevo.
16 Geertz G. The Politics of Meaning. *The Interpretation of Cultures.* New York: Basic Books, 1973, pp. 312–26.
17 Sontag S. *Illness As Metaphor and AIDS and Its Metaphors.* New York: Anchor, 1990.
18 Altman D. *AIDS and the New Puritanism.* London: Pluto Press, 1986.
19 For example, Kubler-Ross E. *On Death and Dying.* Collier Books, 1997.
20 For example, see Kleinman A, Good B. *Culture and Depression. Studies in the Anthropology and Cross-Cultural Psychiatry of Affect and Disorder.* Berkeley: University of California Press, 1985.

21 Lawrence C. Definite and Material: Coronary Thrombosis and Cardiologists in the 1920s. In Rosenberg CE, Golden J eds. *Framing Disease: Studies in Cultural History.* New Brunswick: Rutgers University Press, 1992, pp. 50–84.
22 See for example Young A. *The Harmony of Illusions. Inventing Post-Traumatic Stress Disorder.* Princeton, NJ: Princeton University Press, 1995.
23 Aronowitz RA. 'From Myalgic Encephalitis to Yuppie Flu: A History of Chronic Fatigue Syndromes. In Rosenberg CE, Golden J eds. *Framing Disease: Studies in Cultural History.* New Brunswick: Rutgers University Press, 1992, pp. 155–84.
24 Kleinman A. *The Illness Narratives. Suffering, Healing & the Human Condition.* New York: Basic Books, 1988.
25 Sontag S. *Illness as Metaphor.* Harmondsworth, Middlesex: Penguin Books, 1983, p. 7.
26 Sacks O. *A leg to stand on.* New York: Summit Books, 1984, p. 81.
27 For example, see case studies in Kleinman A. *The Illness Narratives.* New York: Basic Books, 1988.
28 Hacking I. *The Taming of Chance.* Cambridge: Cambridge University Press, 1990.

Illness stories

3 The median isn't the message

Stephen Jay Gould

My life has recently intersected, in a most personal way, two of Mark Twain's famous quips. One I shall defer to the end of this essay. The other (sometimes attributed to Disraeli) identifies three species of mendacity, each worse than the one before – lies, damned lies, and statistics.

Consider the standard example of stretching truth with numbers – a case quite relevant to my story. Statistics recognises different measures of an "average", or central, tendency. The mean represents our usual concept of an overall average – add up the items and divide them by the number of sharers (100 candy bars collected for five kids next Hallowe'en will yield 20 for each in a fair world). The *median,* a different measure of central tendency, is the halfway point. If I line up five kids by height, the median child is shorter than two and taller than the other two (who might have trouble getting their mean share of the candy). A politician in power might say with pride, "The mean income of our citizens is $15 000 per year." The leader of the opposition might retort, "But half our citizens make less than $10 000 per year." Both are right, but neither cites a statistic with impassive objectivity. The first invokes a mean, the second a median. (Means are higher than medians in such cases because one millionaire may outweigh hundreds of poor people in setting a mean, but can balance only one mendicant in calculating a median.)

The larger issue that creates a common distrust or contempt for statistics is more troubling. Many people make an unfortunate and invalid separation between heart and mind, or feeling and intellect. In some contemporary traditions, abetted by attitudes stereotypically centered upon Southern California, feelings are exalted as more "real" and the only proper basis for action, while intellect gets short shrift as a hang-up of outmoded elitism. Statistics, in this absurd dichotomy, often becomes the symbol of the enemy. As Hilaire Belloc wrote, "Statistics are the triumph of the quantitative

29

method, and the quantitative method is the victory of sterility and death."

This is a personal story of statistics, properly interpreted, as profoundly nurturant and life-giving. It declares holy war on the downgrading of intellect by telling a small story to illustrate the utility of dry, academic knowledge about science. Heart and head are focal points of one body, one personality.

In July 1982, I learned that I was suffering from abdominal mesothelioma, a rare and serious cancer usually associated with exposure to asbestos. When I revived after surgery, I asked my first question of my doctor and chemotherapist: "What is the best technical literature about mesothelioma?" She replied, with a touch of diplomacy (the only departure she has ever made from direct frankness), that the medical literature contained nothing really worth reading.

Of course, trying to keep an intellectual away from literature works about as well as recommending chastity to *Homo sapiens,* the sexiest primate of all. As soon as I could walk, I made a beeline for Harvard's Countway medical library and punched mesothelioma into the computer's bibliographic search program. An hour later, surrounded by the latest literature on abdominal mesothelioma, I realized with a gulp why my doctor had offered that humane advice. The literature couldn't have been more brutally clear: mesothelioma is incurable, with a median mortality of only 8 months after discovery. I sat stunned for about 15 minutes, then smiled and said to myself .... so that's why they didn't give me anything to read. Then my mind started to work again, thank goodness.

If a little learning could ever be a dangerous thing, I had encountered a classic example. Attitude clearly matters in fighting cancer. We don't know why (from my old-style materialistic perspective, I suspect that mental states feed back upon the immune system). But match people with the same cancer for age, class, health, and socioeconomic status, and, in general, those with positive attitudes, with a strong will and purpose for living, with commitment to struggle, and with an active response to aiding their own treatment and not just a passive acceptance of anything doctors say, tend to live longer. A few months later I asked Sir Peter Medawar, my personal scientific guru and a Nobelist in immunology what the best prescription for success against cancer might be. "A sanguine personality", he replied. Fortunately (since one can't reconstruct oneself at short notice and for a definite purpose), I am, if anything, even-tempered and confident in just this manner.

Hence the dilemma for humane doctors: since attitude matters so critically, should such a sombre conclusion be advertised, especially since few people have sufficient understanding of statistics to evaluate what the statements really mean? From years of experience with the small-scale evolution of Bahamian land snails treated quantitatively, I have developed this technical knowledge – and I am convinced that it played a major role in saving my life. Knowledge is indeed power, as Francis Bacon proclaimed.

The problem may be briefly stated: what does "median mortality of 8 months" signify in our vernacular? I suspect that most people, without training in statistics, would read such a statement as "I will probably be dead in 8 months" – the very conclusion that must be avoided, both because this formulation is false, and because attitude matters so much.

I was not, of course, overjoyed, but I didn't read the statement in this vernacular way either. My technical training enjoined a different perspective on "8 months median mortality". The point may seem subtle, but the consequences can be profound. Moreover, this perspective embodies the distinctive way of thinking in my own field of evolutionary biology and natural history.

We still carry the historical baggage of a Platonic heritage that seeks sharp essences and definite boundaries. (Thus we hope to find an unambiguous "beginning of life" or "definition of death", although nature often comes to us as irreducible continua.) This Platonic heritage, with its emphasis on clear distinctions and separated immutable entities, leads us to view statistical measures of central tendency wrongly, indeed opposite to the appropriate interpretation in our actual world of variation, shadings, and continua. In short, we view means and medians as hard "realities", and the variation that permits their calculation as a set of transient and imperfect measurements of this hidden essence. If the median is the reality and variation around the median just a device for calculation, then "I will probably be dead in 8 months" may pass as a reasonable interpretation.

But all evolutionary biologists know that variation itself is nature's only irreducible essence. Variation is the hard reality, not a set of imperfect measures for a central tendency. Means and medians are the abstractions. Therefore, I looked at the mesothelioma statistics quite differently – and not only because I am an optimist who tends to see the doughnut instead of the hole, but primarily because I know that variation itself is the reality. I had to place myself amidst the variation.

When I learned about the 8-month median, my first intellectual reaction was: fine, half the people will live longer; now what are my chances of being in that half? I read for a furious and nervous hour and concluded, with relief: damned good. I possessed every one of the characteristics conferring a probability of longer life: I was young; my disease had been recognised in a relatively early stage; I would receive the nation's best medical treatment. I had the world to live for; I knew how to read the data properly and not despair.

Another technical point then added even more solace. I immediately recognised that the distribution of variation about the 8-month median would almost surely be what statisticians call "right-skewed". (In a symmetrical distribution, the profile of variation to the left of the central tendency is a mirror image of variation to the right. Skewed distributions are asymmetrical, with variation stretching out more in one direction than the other – left-skewed if extended to the left, right-skewed if stretched out to the right.) The distribution of variation had to be right-skewed, I reasoned. After all, the left of the distribution contains an irrevocable lower boundary of zero (since mesothelioma can only be identified at death or before). Thus, little space exists for the distribution's lower (or left) half – it must be scrunched up between zero and 8 months. But the upper (or right) half can extend out for years and years, even if nobody ultimately survives. The distribution must be right-skewed, and I needed to know how long the extended tail ran – for I had already concluded that my favorable profile made me a good candidate for the right half of the curve.

The distribution was, indeed, strongly right-skewed, with a long tail (however small) that extended for several years above the 8-month median. I saw no reason why I shouldn't be in that small tail, and I breathed a very long sigh of relief. My technical knowledge had helped. I had read the graph correctly. I had asked the right question and found the answers. I had obtained, in all probability, that most precious of all possible gifts in the circumstances – substantial time. I didn't have to stop and immediately follow Isaiah's injunction to Hezekiah: "set thine house in order: for thou shalt die, and not live." I would have time to think, to plan, and to fight.

One final point about statistical distributions. They apply only to a prescribed set of circumstances – in this case to survival with mesothelioma under conventional modes of treatment. If circumstances change, the distribution may alter. I was placed on an experimental protocol of treatment and, if fortune holds, will be in the first cohort of a new distribution with high median and a right tail extending to death by natural causes at advanced old age.

It has become, in my view, a bit too trendy to regard the acceptance of death as something tantamount to intrinsic dignity. Of course I agree with the preacher of Ecelesiastes that there is a time to love and a time to die – and when my skein runs out I hope to face the end calmly and in my own way. For most situations, however, I prefer the more martial view that death is the ultimate enemy – and I find nothing reproachable in those who rage mightily against the dying of the light.

The swords of battle are numerous, and none more effective than humour. My death was announced at a meeting of my colleagues in Scotland and I almost experienced the delicious pleasure of reading my obituary penned by one of my best friends (the so-and-so got suspicious and checked; he too is a statistician, and didn't expect to find me so far out on the left tail). Still, the incident provided my first good laugh after the diagnosis. Just think, I almost got to repeat Mark Twain's most famous line of all: "the reports of my death are greatly exaggerated".

Post script

Since writing this, my death has actually been reported in two European magazines, 5 years apart. Fama volat (and lasts a long time). I squawked very loudly both times and demanded a retraction; I guess I just don't have Mr Twain's *savoir faire*.

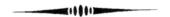

4 The night my life changed

Robert McCrum

No one will ever know exactly what happened in my head one summer night 3 years ago, but probably it went something like this. First, a surreptitious clot began to form deep inside one of my cerebral arteries, cutting off the blood supply to the one organ in the body that, next to the heart, is greediest for blood. Eventually, perhaps some hours later, the clot burst in the right side of my brain – an uncontrolled "bleed" that would result in irreversible destruction of the brain tissue. I was unaware of this cerebral drama; all I knew was that when I went to bed I had a raging headache, and then, the next morning, I could hardly move. Overnight, I had suffered what a specialist called a "right-hemisphere haemorrhagic infarct", or what the world knows as "a stroke" – a word whose Old English origin connotes "a blow" and "a calamity".

It's a calamity that befalls some 100,000 Britons each year, of whom about a third will die immediately. But when it happened to me, I was completely ignorant of the affliction.

It was just another Saturday morning when I found myself in bed, alone and unable to get up at home in Islington, north London. My wife, Sarah Lyall, a journalist, was in San Francisco. It was odd to be on my own and odder still to be so helpless, but I was in no pain, and, in retrospect, I realise that I was barely half conscious. Downstairs, the grandfather clock was chiming the hour: 8 o'clock. I could see that beyond the heavy maroon curtains it was a lovely day. I was supposed to drive to Cambridge to visit my parents. So, it was time to get up. But I could not move my left side. My body had become a dead weight of nearly 15 stone. I thrashed about in bed trying to sit upright, and wishing Sarah were with me. I experienced no anxiety – just irritation and puzzlement.

I have relived this moment, when my life divided into "old" and "new", a thousand times. Strangely, I had felt ready for a change, though I could not say what kind. I was 42. For 17 years, I'd burned the candle at both ends and earned my living as the editorial director of the publishers Faber & Faber, working with writers such as Kazuo Ishiguro and Milan Kundera; I also write fiction and have sometimes combined this with freelance journalism in troubled parts of the world.

Mentally, I wore a flak jacket and jeans under my yuppie suit, and I liked to think I was more at home on the road than in the chic, heartless salons of London. Indeed, on the evening of my collapse, I'd done something I now think of as typical of my "old" life: I'd gone out for dinner at the Ivy, a restaurant in Covent Garden with Kathy Robbins, a literary agent. Before setting off, I'd swallowed a couple of Nurofen for the headache that had been troubling me all day. At the Ivy, I ordered champagne. (In that life, a glass of champagne would dispel most troubles.) But by the time Kathy and I were sitting with our coffees, I still had a headache and I remember yawning with unaccountable weariness, wondering why, after only two glasses, my speech was so muddy and indistinct. My American Express receipt shows that I paid for our meal at 22:38; my signature was steady. But something was not quite right. I said goodnight to Kathy and, desperate to be home, hailed a taxi.

When we reached Islington, my legs felt like lead, and I was walking like a deep-sea diver. I was plainly unwell, but my symptoms were unfamiliar. So I turned to that sovereign English remedy: a cup of tea. Downstairs in the kitchen, I listened to a cheery message from Sarah on our answering machine. It included a hotel number to call, but, feeling extraordinarily tired, I decided to wait until morning and climbed upstairs to bed. When a stroke occurs, the body experiences a colossal disturbance of its innate sensory equilibrium. I was conscious and alert (I thought), but my limbs were not responding. My recollection of the first phase of the morning is disconnected and hallucinatory.

With difficulty, I rolled to the edge of our big brass bed. Then I was falling heavily to the floor, dragged over the edge of the bed by the dead weight of my left side. I was shocked and dismayed, and my first thought was to telephone for help. There was a phone on the bedside table, but that was now out of reach. So there I was: naked and cut off. I suppose I passed out, because when I came to again the street was noisier and busier, and the sun was high. When the telephone rang briefly, maddeningly, and stopped, I knew that the answering machine would be clicking into action. Up here in the bedroom, it was out of earshot.

Time blurred. When I heard the clock chime again, it was three. Lying on the floor, I became obsessed by my missed rendezvous with my parents. At times, bizarrely persuaded by the remaining strength in my right side, I imagined hobbling across the street to my car, somehow driving with one arm. I was like a rat on a wheel, revolving desperate escape plans. Then the phone rang again. Somehow, I knew I had to get to the phone on the floor of the living room. With what I now see must have been an extraordinary effort, I dragged myself over the carpet to the head of the stairs.

Here, reaching out to the bannister, which, fortunately, was on my right side, I pulled myself forward over the top step. Again, my dead weight took control, and I found I was sliding helplessly and painfully head first down the carpeted stairs to the mezzanine landing, where I had a Borrower's-eye view of my library of first editions. I vividly remember this part of the day. It was dawning on me that I was no longer the person I'd been 24 hours ago. From time to time, my thoughts, such as they were, would be interrupted by the phone. I thought I could detect the faint whir and click of the machine and then Sarah's voice. I was terribly frustrated. I wanted to call out: "Darling, I'm here. Please come and help me."

As evening drew on, I decided I had to try the descent down the final flight of stairs to the living room. This time, I controlled my weight with my right hand on the bannister, inching head-first down to the hallway. It was gloomy, and pleasantly cool. The clock, whose chimes had punctuated my day, was ticking steadily nearby. More squirming, and I was in the sitting room – and there, across the carpet, was the phone. I felt like a pioneer who, crossing the Rockies, finally arrives in California. British Telecom records show that I called my parents – it never occurred to me to call Emergency – at 19:53. Apparently, I told my anxious mother that I could not move. Now things began to happen fast. When the phone rang again, it was my brother Stephen. He and his fiancee, Emily, were on their way and had phoned the police. I heard a siren outside and then a voice through the letterbox. I replied, with difficulty: "No, I can't open the door." Another siren; the sound of splitting wood. I remember worrying about being naked, but exhaustion was stronger than modesty.

Soon, I was propped up in the ambulance. I took Emily's hand and felt her answering squeeze. I was so happy. I was with my family. I was going to the hospital, I had survived.

My doctor, Andrew Lees advised me to think of the bleed as a kind of bruise; over time, the scavenging macrophage cells would literally eat up the damage to the cerebral tissue, leaving that part of my brain scarred. An early scan located the bleed, a menacing black blot, deep in the brain. The sinister stain would gradually shrink and fade, but, despite this brilliant pictorial representation, I am no nearer a reliable explanation of why the stroke occurred. Indeed, about 40% of strokes are unexplained. This is unnerving for patients and doctors alike. When my rehabilitation specialist, Dr Richard Greenwood, confessed that doctors are quite ignorant about the brain, it was oddly comforting.

I had to face up to the slow process of recovery, which, in the case of a stroke, offers a moving target: one is imperceptibly getting better. I had also to learn to adjust, and to wait. Before all this, I could slip across the street to post a letter in the time it takes to type a sentence. For about a year, I had to raise myself from my chair, find my walking stick, limp to the front door (say, 3 minutes), negotiate the steps to the street, and make my way to the corner (roughly 5 minutes), and then hobble back and collapse on the sofa, as though I had just run a marathon. I used to be known for the impressionistic speed with which I could do things, but I have now become friends with slowness, both as a concept and as a way of life. Sometimes it is difficult to admit that the stroke was an irrevocable event in my personal history. To admit that I have been scared and lonely is as difficult as it is to admit that I can sometimes feel a profound anger toward the world that has done this to me.

Sometimes, I think, perhaps I am dreaming. Occasionally, I even say out loud: "Am I dreaming? Did this really happen?" But no, I am not dreaming. Even though I am much better now, I am changed forever.

This is an edited extract from *My year off: rediscovering life after a stroke* by Robert McCrum, London: Picador, 1998. We are grateful to the author and publisher for kind permission to reproduce this excerpt.

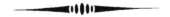

5 The good bleed guide

Donald Bateman

It was about 1920, when my son Donald was at the crawling around stage, that he cut the skin between his upper lip and gum and bled heavily. I had to take him to hospital and they stitched it up several times and told me that he seemed to be "a bleeder".

He had bad episodes with tooth extraction and had to go into Leeds General Infirmary, where the only treatment was repeated stitching of the gums. I was then told that my son had "spongy gums". When I pointed out that my brother and uncle had a similar condition and I thought it was something more serious I was told that "they must have spongy gums also". Not until he was about 11 years old was the word "haemophilia" ever mentioned.

I remember once when he was in hospital, very ill, and they could not stop him bleeding and I interrupted several times to tell them that I thought I could do better myself with dressings and pressure. They seemed to be so anxious about things that they let me take over myself at the bedside. He must have been bad or they would not have let me go near his bed! It was after this episode that I heard a nurse warn a doctor to "beware of his mother for she interferes". I felt glad that I did, for mothers worry about their children when they are ill and suffering.

It would have been helpful if doctors had given me any information. The fact that they did not do so led me to believe that they knew nothing about the subject of the blood. For example, we could never understand why Donald bruised so easily and so heavily. When I took him to see our doctor with bad and ugly bruised areas he simply told me to apply hot poultices and then witch hazel. We had to be careful about using the doctor for each visit cost 2/6 including a bottle of medicine and it was 3/6 if he visited us. We paid cash but for those who could not afford to he employed a collector who went round collecting 2d or 3d a time. We were all right with the hospital and ambulances because Dad paid a penny a week to the Workpeople's Hospital Fund in Leeds by stoppage from his wages.

It was about 1947 when a hospital first asked me to provide a 'family tree' showing relatives who bled badly.

It would have been such a great help to mothers if doctors had been able to tell them something about the illness but they were all tin gods on a pedestal and never told us anything. They seemed to think they were doing you a favour if they spoke to you at all.

Verbatim transcript of account by Mrs Emily Bateman, mother of the author, recorded on a tape dated July 7th 1973, when she was 80 years old.

The history of medicine is officially recorded by its practitioners, or researchers, and not its victims. The sick, like the poor, leave few archives behind them.

There are areas where the ignorance of bedside practitioners has led to monumental errors. The elite position of medical doctors before World War II gave them an immunity from criticism. Once the average GP had qualified, his (almost invariably male) knowledge was deemed to last him throughout his career. The elitism of medical practitioners deterred them from accepting evidence often spread out for their examination by patients.

A patient with a chronic condition may have more experience (subjectively) than many of the practitioners treating him. No better example exists than that of haemophilia, of which I am one of the select 5000 in Britain. Born in 1919, I span the spectrum from total ignorance and wrong treatment, to solving the problem with safe (I hope!) Factor VIII.

I owe my survival in boyhood and youth less to the medical profession than the innate good sense of my working class, socialist, Quaker parents. I have the classical pattern of sex-linked inheritance; my mother's brother and her uncle were haemophiliacs, but this was accepted as evidence by doctors only in the later 1930s. When a baby,[1] I cut the skin inside the upper lip, the frenum, rich in blood vessels and a vulnerable locality. My first stay in hospital and repeated stitching I do not remember, but I was 10 years old when given the authentic term "bleeder".

A learned journal of the time advised doctors: "Bleeders with means should take up some learned profession and if they are students, duelling should be forbidden."[2] There were precious few people with means in Holbeck, where I grew up, and duelling was not part of our culture. The advice was certainly well taken by the Spanish Royal family who had mattresses on their lawns and playrooms, and padded the tree-trunks for a play area for their haemophiliac son. Whenever as a boy I had bad bleeds and massive painful haematomas from tumbling around, my mother was advised to treat them with a hot poultice. Today, the treatment is to pack it with ice! If you think I exaggerate, there is ample evidence that the recommended treatment did not change for the next 40 years. A mother, Mrs Norma Guy, revealed in the *Haemophilia Journal*[3] that in the late 1960s "I was told by my GP to apply a hot kaolin poultice and keep it warm".

There was an assumption in "respectable circles" that the condition arose from close inter-marriage or incestuous relationships. The appearance of the condition in various crowned heads of Europe with Queen Victoria as the transmitting agent were to blame for this. The name haemophilia surfaced in 1854. This ties in with Victoria and the first recognition of inherited transmission. Medical textbooks credit it to a treatise by Hopff in 1823,[4] and the name was used by medical doctors only between themselves. In sparse conversations with patients they referred to them as "bleeders". They had two languages, one for professional purposes and one for the sub-culture of patients. As a boy, doctors spoke to me as a "bleeder", a laughter-provoking term I resented, and I became part of the general conspiracy to hide the condition. The label was worse than the complaint; it conditioned one into a lowering of self esteem. The correct medical term would have given it some authentic respectability, but it was 1951 before the Haemophilia Society popularised the official name.

Medical ignorance and a refusal to accept my mother's evidence in the 1920s, created a situation where, when I was bleeding profusely from the loss of milk teeth, a hospital doctor told her "Your boy suffers from spongy gums". He saw me again, after I had been bleeding for another couple of weeks. My mother (with the persistence which often proved to be my best protective shield) pointed out that her brother and uncle both shared the same condition and she was told that they too must have enjoyed "spongy gums"; it was an inherited tendency. After remarking that she did not have the same complaint, she was off-loaded as a trouble-maker. Anyone with an unknown or persistent problem was a nuisance to the average general hospital and its casualty department, yet such people could have been a rich mine of information. From this incident alone a correct diagnosis of my condition could have been made.

When young I broke my thigh and spent an eternity in hospital. Contemporary thought is that children can suffer long-term psychological damage from being separated from their mothers at times of stress. My parents were allowed to visit me only once per calendar month! Investigations pioneered by James Robertson on children evacuated during the war, developed modern thinking where mothers can be provided with a bed in the hospital and contact maintained with a sick child.[5] I was distraught about long stays in hospitals, even though my parents did everything to try and make me feel I was not forgotten. The anguish came from knowing that the medical people were mystified by my condition and had not the slightest idea how to treat it. Ignorance can be all-pervasive. I already knew that they knew … nothing.

As a youngster I experienced this strange and alienating condition with panic and few resources for combating it. After a tooth extraction, I was afraid to go to sleep in case I suffocated from the masses of coagulated blood filling my throat, nose and mouth in my rather tentative cat-napping. Hospital attempts at person-to-person blood transfusions provoked massive rigors at a time when knowledge of blood typing was limited. My terror was equalled by that, 40 years later, of Mrs Guy's son. As she subsequently related, "He became quite scared of doctors – what they called a white coat syndrome. They had to remove their white coats before he would let any of them near to him".[3]

The terror which consumed me in boyhood about hospitals was partly a reflection of medical attitudes. Doctors assumed that I was devoid of comprehension, but young boys are quick in perception. Medical ignorance heightened my fears. Some kind of education could have prevented the kind of alienation which a young haemophiliac can so easily develop against himself.

In hospital, like a prisoner in solitary confinement, I had little contact with the outside world. Young children were known only by their surnames. There was no promise of good conduct remission or parole as there is in prison. There was no effort to provide education, and there were no telephones or visitors, other than distant and aloof parsons who even harangued young boys about the state of their immortal souls. Such visitations increased the terror, as may be appreciated. When in 1991 I had a bad internal bleed after a knock on the hand (which after a few hours resembled a boxing glove), I sought Factor VIII for the first time in about 8 years, having refused such treatment – because of HIV. The young hospital doctor who pumped the elixir into me said "You must have had bumps like this as a boy. What was the treatment?" I could only tell him that it would have been encased in plaster and my mother would have held the other hand.

In the long chronicle of cures-which-failed, Russell's Viper Venom must take pride of place. This vile extract from an Indian snake was painted on to a tooth socket – very bitter and acidic.

When applied to gums, or tongue, the blood curdled into a horrible precipitate. The clot was an acidic, congealed mass which grew in the mouth until the patient was in danger of choking. Very rarely was any progress made at the first attempt and the patient endured repeated treatment. For tooth extraction a plastic splint was made, venom on gauze inserted, the mouth shut and bandaging applied round the jaws and top of the head to keep the whole ghastly creation in place. Modern technology intervened and it was developed as a mediaeval Scolds' Bridle with a headpiece, rubber or leather straps, and a ratchet to hold the appliance in place. Venom was also used on open cuts and wounds. It was a valiant attempt at coping with a problem, but all the R&D work was going into the wrong aspect of the condition.

In the obituary notices for Professor Robert Gwyn Macfarlane he is credited with first extracting and using Russell's Viper Venom on a haemophiliac in July 1934.[6] I was an early recipient in Leeds General Infirmary and though praise is rightly heaped upon the originator, no-one ever mentions the horrors bestowed upon the patients! We were experimental subjects. My faded memories of the experience are due not to old age but general weakness in the relevant period. A major problem was that the patient in pre NHS days was never told what was being done to him. He was an object to be talked about but never with. Doctors would discuss the condition of a patient across the two sides of the bed as if it was empty. The patient and his fears were, it seemed, ignored.

Medical ignorance has much to answer for – and the patient paid the price. There has been insufficient recognition of the price which haemophiliac mothers pay. As the carriers, many of them have a burden of guilt, yet in the past felt powerless to do anything about the problem. Mrs Guy has emphasised her sense of guilt: "He was in pain because of me ... this feeling of guilt still haunts me".[3]

In July 1947 I entered hospital in the long vacation to have three teeth extracted. It is no exaggeration to say that it almost killed me. As preliminary treatment I had to swallow massive doses of calcium tablets nightly for a couple of weeks before admission. The night before the extraction I had 20. They were of course valueless other than in producing acute constipation; I ended up a thoroughly bloody mess in intensive care.

In 1962 I had an even more painful and hazardous dental experience lasting 4 weeks; it took me as long again to recover. I was given a penicillin injection into my left thigh muscle, despite my warnings from previous episodes. This was a disaster for I bled heavily internally; I fainted and my leg had to be plaster-casted yet again. I must be the only man ever to go into hospital to have three teeth out and be discharged on crutches! Liberal coatings of Viper Venom brought little success and the damage to my leg was profound. A cardinal rule in modern treatment today is "Do not use intra-muscular injections at any time with haemophiliacs" and modern haematology textbooks specifically warn against the dangers of such treatment. My tender and painful thigh is a legacy of hospital ignorance for any doctor should have been aware of the hazard with intra-muscular injections – I warned them myself but to no avail. I now walk with a stick. In 1962 my GP gave me their report of this episode, which is full of inaccuracies – even the dates of my entry and exit are wrong!

It is only 20 years ago that I visited a strange hospital after a bleed and presented the Casualty Officer with my Haemophiliac Green card. He took a puzzled look at it and said: "How long have you been a haemophiliac?". A fellow sufferer assures me that he has heard of a similar occurrence within the last 5 years.

After a whole series of unsuccessful nostrums, Cryoprecipitate, rich in the clotting agents Factor VIII and fibrinogen, was the first major breakthrough in treatment of haemophilia. It required a great volume for treatment and garden-syringe injections of the near-frozen solution rushed straight to my head with unpleasant side effects.

The advent of Factor VIII should have been our life-giving elixir, but the HIV story has been well-chronicled.[7] Although the first haemophiliac to die of AIDS did so in Bristol, I was miraculously reprieved even though I had been transfused with Factor VIII at about the same time as the victim. For 7 years I then refused Factor VIII because biochemist colleagues of mine had warned me of its dangers. If it was obvious to me then it should have been so to all those connected with the haematology service, yet 1500 haemophiliacs became HIV positive and many died. In 1984 I was knocked down by a car and shipped into hospital by ambulance. I refused Factor VIII and was then told to make my own way home for I had "refused treatment". Thank God I did .... I am HIV negative and many friends from that 7-year period are dead or HIV positive.

My hairiest period was when I was being tested at regular intervals for several years for "HIV positivity". Other patients, whom I knew, tested positive and my transfusion dates were close to theirs. I knew for a period what it was like to be in the condemned cell awaiting a possible reprieve. This is the great tragedy. Our life-saving treatment killed so many of my friends.

The greatest scandal was the initial denial of any linkage between AIDS and Factor VIII products. We were bulldozed into accepting Factor VIII, even though later, the Government said "They sought medication – tough luck". I was actually sent for twice "for counselling" because I refused Factor VIII in the vital period of risk.

I am a great survivor; at the age of 78 I have achieved an exalted state of semi-normality. I lead an active life ... except that for almost 20 years I have had hepatitis C from blood products. This in itself is a high penalty. There is no free lunch; we have paid too high a price.

This article is an extract (edited by the author), reproduced from The good bleed guide: a patient's story. *Social History of Medicine* 1994:115–33.

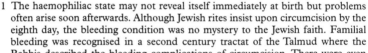

1 The haemophiliac state may not reveal itself immediately at birth but problems often arise soon afterwards. Although Jewish rites insist upon circumcision by the eighth day, the bleeding condition was no mystery to the Jewish faith. Familial bleeding was recognised in a second century tractat of the Talmud where the Rabbis described the bleeding complications of circumcision. There were even exemptions for Jewish families where the first two sons had experienced bleeding problems at circumcision.
2 Quoted in Massey R, Massey S. *Journey.* 1972 (English edition 1973), pp. 20–1.
3 *The Haemophilia Society Bulletin,* No. 4, 1991.
4 Ingram CIG. The history of haemophilia. *J Clin Pathology* 1976; **29**: 469–79.
5 James Robertson who worked at the Tavistock Clinic had an enormous influence upon the way in which children are treated, particularly in hospital. He was a tireless campaigner for the principle that a mother should be with a sick child as much as possible. He had a great influence on Sir Harry Platt whose report to the Government advocated that mothers should be allowed freely into children's wards. He died in December 1988 and his posthumously published work *Studies Of Very Young Children In Hospital, Fostercare And Institutions* (London, 1989) deals with the subject.
6 Dr Alastair Robb-Smith. "Professor Robert Gwyn Macfarlane CBE MA MD FRCP'. This excellent obituary article published in *The Haemophilia Bulletin* 1987; No.3, pp. 3–5, gives full details of his achievements in Haematology and the date of July 19th 1934 for the first use of Russell's Viper venom. The haemophilia Society honours the man who was its president by awarding a Gold Medal bearing his name to individuals who have made important contributions to the study of the condition.
7 Fee E, Fox DM. *AIDS: the burden of history.* Berkeley: University of California Press, 1988.

6 Stories of dying: therapeutic writing in hospice care

Gillie Bolton

Well, I'm not sure how or where to begin.

Hospice patient

I never knew birds sang in winter until I had cancer.

Cancer patient quoted Pat Pilkington[1]

Verse is for healthy arty-farties. The dying and surgeons use prose.

Peter Reading from 'C'[2]

This last is not true at all; the poet Peter Reading[2] is well known for using outrageousness to make people think. Poetry is peculiarly appropriate to the dying due to its conciseness, brevity, and lyricism. My story, here, however, focuses on the writing of narratives. There are a range of fearful words for the dying, denoted by their initial letter. Reading's C word is one, as is the big G (God); W for Writing is another. "Oh I couldn't do that" a healthy person, and often a dying one, will say.

Yet, in extremis, the dying can find writing a deeply healing activity; just as they wish to hear the word God, and often want to face up to facts about their cancer. Writing ceases to be a frightening activity associated with school, which only clever people or arty-farties can do. It becomes a way of expressing some of their response to the turmoil of change taking place in this last precious bit of their lives. Not all this turmoil is negative: the knowledge of the closeness of death seems to sharpen awareness of the beauties of life. Writing is a perfect way of celebrating these, as well as a way of bringing outside that which is causing pain inside.

45

It all goes round and round in my head, you see. I'm not very good at talking. But the writing - it seemed to get it out there, stopped it going round and round. Now I can see it in writing, I can sort it out more. Reading it out to the group wasn't easy, but it gave me a way of saying something to them which I couldn't say otherwise. I said it in the writing.

Mavis, a hospice patient

Palliative care has a reputation for its holistic attention to patients and their families. Many hospice services have units for day-patients which are also available to in-patients who are sufficiently mobile to join in. Arts and crafts are brought for patients to try their hand; and creative writing has become part of this. The research reported here – a project that aimed to chart the potentially therapeutic power of writing – is part of a move to locate arts and humanities firmly in mainstream medicine and nursing.

Writing promotes healing

Something said and heard can never be unspoken – as we all know from having to live with the things we've yelled in rows. Writing on the other hand is private, a communication with the self, until the patient decides to share it – usually after solitary reflective rereading. Writing is often a staged process of rereading, redrafting and sharing. Unshareable things can therefore be expressed relatively safely in writing.

When the patient is ready, writing can be a supremely effective form of communication with chosen others, offering a lasting record for the self, family, and friends. The creative process of writing is rewarding (often exciting and fun), increasing self confidence and self esteem. Discussions around pieces of writing may be deep and significant. A writing group can be a relatively safe, supportive, yet challenging environment for patients to explore and share vital elements within their changing, sometimes joyful, but often depressing or frightening world.

Several patients in my study found that writing a narrative of their fears, anxieties, anger or bewilderment helped them to face, understand, and to an extent, come to terms with these emotions. The staff reported that this reduction in stress sometimes helped relieve their symptoms. One patient could not accept she had cancer, and was in great turmoil within herself. She dictated her writing, as her hands had been affected by the treatment, sitting looking away from me, talking and talking with no reference to my presence. Tears streamed down her face, and she said she had not cried since her diagnosis over a year previously. She blessed the writing over and over for allowing her to face the diagnosis and to express fearful thoughts such as her desire to commit suicide. Many patients were grateful for the release of tears which a rereading of their writing allowed them.

Another patient, very near death, was in such great distress, the staff were unable to console him. He wrote for a mere 15 minutes – almost unintelligibly. But he wrote the names of his first partner, and those of their children. Having written, he was then able to talk about them, ask to see them, say goodbye and to express sorrow about what had passed between them. When I called in the next day he lay there quiet, looked up at me and smiled. "Happy", was all he said: "happy, happy".

Writing is essentially different from talking. Talking and thinking may dissipate or change like Chinese whispers. Writing helps patients work on things. It stays there on the page in the same form; it doesn't go away unless and until it is worked on again (next day/ year). It can create pathways to memories, feelings, and thoughts patients do not always know that they have, enabling them to discover, explore, clarify, and make connections with the present. Issues, ideas, inspirations they are aware of, but seem problematic or hard to communicate, can thereby be expressed.

Patients sometimes have an initial fear or inhibition about starting to write. But my experience is that this melts away very quickly once they start, and have begun to realise the benefits; and once they understand they needn't worry about spelling, grammar, form, or writing a perfect piece. Writing is like most of life – a narrative all muddly middle without the neat beginnings and endings of fiction. I always encourage patients to begin from where they are – the middle. This is writing which is primarily for the writer; though it also has great power to communicate effectively with others.

An increasing number of publications in Britain recognise the power of this sort of writing.[3-7] Eleanor Nesbitt has written in *Linkup* about her experiences of writing as a cancer sufferer, encouraging others to do the same[8]:

> I felt a strong inner compulsion to record what I was going through and made sure I had plenty of paper and pens in hospital. Even in the dark, one sleepless night, I wrote blindly, capturing images and fleeting thoughts without the fear that they would have evaporated by the morning medicine round.

I would rather throw them away in the cold light of day than feel I had let something precious and fleeting slip past irrevocably. Both writing and reading my diary entries have clarified my feelings and ideas.

Background to writing in the hospice

Writers (poets, novelists, playwrights, etc.) have known for a very long time that writing is good for you. Yet, unlike the other arts (art, music, drama), it is not an established therapy in Britain. In America there are scriptotherapy and bibliotherapy, and therapeutic writing is used in psychotherapy (the literature is extensive – for example see [17]). There is randomised control trial evidence from America for the effectiveness of writing in certain situations (e.g. [18-20]). In these trials, writing about traumatic incidents led to fewer self-reported days of sickness and physician visits over a 6-month period, improved cellular immune function, and increased positive moods and exam grades.[18] But there have as yet been no controlled trials of this kind of work in Britain, and we are hoping to find funding to mount one.[33]

In Britain, writers have undertaken residencies in hospices for many years, as they have in hospitals, prisons, etc. Dominic McLoughlin ran successful workshops at St Christopher's day unit in London for 6 years. For him, as for many other writers-in-residence, "to promote an enjoyment of literature"[21, 22] is a main aim; expressed therapeutic work with patients is outside their remit.

Jane Eisenhauer was one of the pioneers in this field in the UK, clearly very successfully, at St Joseph's Hospice in Hackney.[23] As well as detailing the benefits of her work to the patients, David Frampton (consultant physician) has commented that reading patients' writing can help health professionals and clergy to work more effectively and sensitively in this area.

Lynne Alexander has written about her work at Sobell House, Oxford,[24] and at St Johns Hospice, Lancaster.[25] Lynne describes herself as having "cobbled together" the poems in the Sobell House collection; this is similar to John Killick's description of his work with dementia sufferers where he has created and published[26] poetry drawn from recorded conversations with patients. John Killick has been writer-in-residence with Westminster Health Care since 1992, helping patients to express themselves. He says insights, however fragmentary, can be gained into the minds of these sufferers, and that this can provide valuable communications not only with carers, relatives and friends, but also with those who seek to understand the nature of the illness.[27]

The role of writing in palliative care is increasing. There are groups and anthologies now in many hospices. The Marie Curie Poets publish their work;[28] Joanna Drazba's poetry collection,[29] published posthumously, has made her something of an emblematic figure in Polish hospice circles. In Australia, Elizabeth Mosely and Tarja Ahokas have published a poetry and painting account of their "healing journey" through "grief, fear, anxiety and the myriad other emotions".[30] Geraldine Monk has contributed very successfully as a writer on the staff of St Lukes, Sheffield.[31] The Christie Hospital, Manchester, publishes a regular anthology;[32] here is the beginning and end of Celia Jones' contribution:

> Word painting
> Where flowers of the wild grow free among grasses
> and bee hives nestle with lichen-barked fruit trees,
> where bluebells and primroses mingle with violets,
> this garden's a tangle of colour and scent.
> ...
>
> And here, at a small wooden table beneath the window,
> she imagines another tangle of colour and scent
> as she paints her garden of words.
>
> *Celia M Jones*

My own experience in this field draws upon work I undertook at Ashgate Hospice, Chesterfield as a pilot project set up by the Palliative Medicine Section of Sheffield University, to study the potential of therapeutic writing in palliative care. Following previous experience in primary care[3 9–11] and work over many years training therapists and counsellors to use writing as an element of their practice,[12 13] I offered writing to in-patients and day-patients one day a week for 6 months. My experience also builds upon work teaching creative writing to English undergraduates at Sheffield Hallam University, and to unemployed people in the residential setting of Northern College.[14–16] Through this work, it became apparent to me that what really engaged students was not the form of the writing (sonnet for example) but, for personal developmental reasons, its content.

Some stories of stories

Mavis made her comment (quoted above) about writing preventing things from going round and round in her head to the

Ashgate Hospice day-unit nurse manager after a group writing session at which she had begun to write her autobiography. Not a verbally articulate person, Mavis had written about her distress at friends abandoning her once they knew she had cancer; her writing examined what their motives might be:

> Strong makes strong, they believe, weak makes weak. But for people like me one has to be strong to conquer our fears. I am weak myself and all I want is to be strong, strong, strong. So who can help me. No-one but myself.

At a later writing session, Norah had absolutely no hesitation about which important memory she wanted to write about. She wrote, and read her writing to us, but was afraid the intensity of her writing meant her first husband was more important to her than her second husband. "No, it just means you have to think about it now for some reason", I responded. She was distressed as she read her piece to us, remembering the way he left her. "It's not surprising you need to think about this now: you didn't say goodbye properly, did you?", I said. "No", she replied simply, folding her paper firmly and putting it in her bag.

One day when Mavis was not there and Norah was having a bath; we started by looking at a piece of writing Dorothy had done the previous week – an expressive piece about feeling trapped by the cancer:

> Let me out
> I seem to have been enclosed
> forever,
> the walls of this prison are closing in
> and I must escape.
>
> How long ago it seems I felt so
> safe
> and secure, but no no longer,
> when did this urge come upon me to escape.
> I twist and turn my body,
> my arms windmilling around my
> head,
> my legs in constant motion,
> God how much longer.
>
> Suddenly through the walls of my
> cell
> I see a light, very pale blue,
> it seems to be so soothing,
> my body absorbs this and I feel more calm.
> What is happening.

The light is getting stronger
I have a feeling of freedom and
comfort
bathed in this warm blue light,
what can it be?
suddenly I have a feeling of wellbeing,
can this last?
I look around me and my eyes
come to rest
on a pale green broken shell;
Has this been my prison for so
long.

Suddenly I am aware of a
presence,
so I feel threatened!!
warm tender hands enfold me
I feel peace,
and this feeling is so good.
Will it last?

I look up and suddenly I am alone again, can this be so?

I look around me
the soothing blue light has faded,
being replaced by a cold grey
light,
I feel my limbs trembling;
my head aches;
I am in despair,
I long for my shell,
to be in my cocoon,
was I safe in there?
my eyes close,
tomorrow is another day;
I can hope!!

Dorothy Lewis

Dorothy read it and we talked about the feelings it gave us. Kath dictated her writing to Val, one of the volunteers: the condition of her hands meant she could not write. She expressed her regret for the past, and her feeling of jealousy of healthy people, adding: "if you put that in it'll make me feel so selfish." She ended with: "I reckon you'd better stop before that page is full of tears".

Kath cried quite a lot with the group that day. She initially was not happy that she had expressed so much in writing, and then cried, feeling she should be brave in front of others. But it gave the other writing group members the opportunity to say self-affirming things to her they would not have been able to say otherwise. They shared their feelings about what the cancer made them feel: depressed, angry, envious, and weepy. Later Kath and several of the others told the day-unit manager how glad they were for the session. Kath died a very short time later.

At her express wish, we read Dorothy's piece to the whole day-unit group. This opened up a great deal of communication (and tears) between patients, and between patients and staff who later felt appreciative of this. Several weeks later, Mavis did some more writing with me. It was a harrowing episode in her autobiography and ended with the word "Amen". When I queried the word, she said it seemed "to end it off properly". I think she wanted to parcel that experience up in the writing, and the Amen was like a tight knot of the string! She talked at length about her previous piece of writing, because doing it had seemed to "bring it home to me". She said she now felt much more in control of her life, and had been able successfully, though painfully, to cut the painful friendships out of her life.

The next time I met the little group, Norah was there in a wheelchair after a protracted spell in hospital. She had done a great deal of thinking as a result of her initial writing about her first husband. Now, her thoughts were all on her operation. She dictated a long piece to Val, the volunteer, about the amputation of her leg. She felt justifiably confident and safe with Val, just as Kath had. Here is an extract:

> My Odd Leg
>
> I'd had problems with my feet for a long time. About 43 years ago I had a bad accident, so I've always had a limp. My left leg had to take my weight always ... . I had problems with ulcers and that, but just accepted that. My husband used to say to me "come on, you odd-legged bugger" and we had a laugh about it ... . Then of course just before Christmas I had at least six months in pain and could hardly walk. They were treating me for ulcers, but my blood wasn't circulating so they decided to take it off ... .
>
> When I woke up I couldn't believe it. I didn't know how much they were taking off – it was such a shock. Mr L explained because of the circulation he'd had to remove a lot.

Norah wanted Val to read her piece to the group, which was a very emotional occasion for all. They had thought and prayed for Norah all the long time she was in hospital; and the group needed to hear the story as much as Norah needed to tell it.

Conclusion

"What the mind represses, the body expresses".[34] Writing seems to be a therapeutically effective way of encouraging those who are near the end of life not to repress, but to express their feelings. The telling of personal stories can provide a powerful means of communicating and communing with fellow patients, professionals, relatives and friends.

Acknowledgments

I would like to acknowledge all the support Tony Bethell, medical director of Ashgate Hospice, and his staff gave to me and the project; the academic, professional and practical assistance of Sam Ahmedzai, Bill Noble, and the Sheffield University Palliative Medicine team; and thank Stephen Rowland. I particularly wish to thank all the patients, who so generously gave me their written permission to quote from their writing.

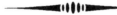

1 Pilkington P. *Summing up of Spirituality and Health Conference*, Durham, Sept/Oct 1997.

2 Reading P. *C: because cowards get cancer too.* London: Secker & Warburg, 1997.

3 Bolton G. *The Therapeutic Potential of Creative Writing: Writing Myself.* London: Jessica Kingsley Publishers, 1998.

4 Jackowska N. *Write for Life: How to Inspire Your Creative Writing.* Shaftsbury: Element Books, 1997.

5 Killick J, Schneider M. *Writing for Self-Discovery.* Shaftsbury: Element Books, 1998.

6 Rainer T. *The New Diary.* London: Angus & Robertson, 1978.

7 Sellers S. *Delighting the Heart.* London: The Women's Press, 1989.

8 Nesbitt E. Writing cancer out of your life. *Linkup* 1997; No 46: pp 7–9.

9 Bolton G. Writing not pills: writing therapy in primary care. In: Hunt C, Samson F eds *The Self on the Page.* London: Jessica Kingsley Publishers, 1998.

10 Bolton G. Buttoned. Writing in Education, *J Nat Assoc Writers Educat* 1997; No 11: pp. 10–14.

11 Bolton G. The Process of Writing gets me in Touch. *Artery* 1996; No. 14: pp. 15–16.

12 Bolton G. Taking the Thinking out of it: Writing, a Therapeutic Space. *J Br Assoc Counsell* 1995; 6: No. 3: 215–18.

13 Bolton G. Just a Bobble Hat: the Story of a Writing as Therapy Training Workshop. Changes, *Int J Psychol Pychother* 1992; 11: No. 1: 37–43.

14 Bolton G, Styles M. There are stories and stories. In: Swindells J ed. *The Uses of Autobiography.* London: Taylor & Francis, 1995.

15 Bolton G. Skills on Call. *Times Educational Supplement*, 13 March 1992.

16 Harrison BT, Bolton G. Realising Through Writing. *J Inst Educat*, Hull University 1990; 96–108.

17 Riordan RJ. Scriptotherapy: therapeutic writing as a counselling adjunct. *J Counsell Devel* 1996; 74: 263–9.

18 Pennebaker JW, Kiecolt-Glaser JK, Glaser, R. Disclosure of traumas and immune function: Health implications for psychotherapy. *J Consult Clin Psychol* 1988; 56: 239–45.

19 Pennebaker JW, Beall SK. Confronting a traumatic event: Toward an understanding of inhibition and disease. *J Abnorm Psychol* 1986; **95**: 274–81.

20 Pennebaker JW, Colder M, Sharp LK. Accelerating the Coping Process. *J Personal Soc Psychol* 1990; **58**: 528–37.

21 McLoughlin D. Creative Writing in Hospice. *Hospice Bulletin: London* 1985; October: pp. 8–9.

22 McLoughlin D. Teaching Writing in a Hospice Day Centre. *Writing in Education, J Natl Assoc Writers Educat* 1987; No. 11: 7–9.

23 Frampton DR. Restoring creativity to the dying patient. *Br Med J* 1986; **293**: No. 6562: 1593–95.

24 Alexander L. In Kaye L, Blee T. *The Arts in Health Care: A Palette of Possibilities*. London: Jessica Kingsley Publishers, 1997.

25 Alexander L ed. *Now I can Tell*. London: Papermac, 1990.

26 Killick J. *You are Words*. London: Hawker Publications, 1997.

27 Killick J. Communicating as if your life depended upon it. In: Heller T. *et al* eds. *Mental Health Matters*. London: Macmillan, 1996, pp. 332–8.

28 Adams PT *et al*. *The Guided Hand*. Liverpool: Sunny Moon Publications, 1997.

29 Drazba J. *Behind the Screen of the Eyelids*. Poznan: Media Rodzina of Poznan, 1997.

30 Mosely E, Ahokas T. *Palette and Pen, A Healing Journey*. Brisbane: Spokespress, 1997.

31 Sutherill C. John's comic relief. *Sheffield Telegraph* 1997; November 29: p. 7.

32 Thwaite J, Ayers D eds. *Patchwork: Poems from The Christie*. Manchester: Christie Hospital, 1997.

33 Bolton G, Ahmedzai S. Project will assess effects of patients writing about their terminal illness on self-perceived quality of life. *Br Med J* 1997; **314**, No. 7092: 1486.

34 Daniel R. *Spirituality and Health Conference*, Durham, Sept/Oct 1997.

7 Narratives of childhood epilepsy: have I got epilepsy or has it got me?

Henrietta Weinbren and Paramjit Gill

Initially we were pretty frightened about it. We didn't know Harriet had epilepsy. We thought initially that she had some kind of dietary disorder and that came out in conversation with [a private doctor] ... so we started to pursue this and we went on looking down this line and of course it was a complete red herring. And then he conducted this very elaborate test and the research was all sent off to California and came back and the Californians said "she has an allergy to everything". So, Harriet went through abandoning all wheat products, abandoning all dairy products, abandoning all soya – we couldn't touch anything – but what was happening was an almost steady starvation ... I had not appreciated what goes on. The relief of that getting a diagnosis was so immense that, huge, I mean it was such a preoccupation, you spent all your time looking at her and wondering what was going on and what she was feeling and you know, I only had that physical manifestation when they did the brain scan, the brain reading – amazing!

Harriet's father

Introduction

Epilepsy is both a medical diagnosis and a social label.[1] [2] Psychosocial consequences include stigma, concealment of the diagnosis, restricted activities and susceptibility to depression.[3] [4] Such problems in adults with epilepsy are associated with the frequency of fits rather than the diagnostic label *per se*, but this may not be the whole story in children.[5] [6] A greater proportion of children with epilepsy show psychosocial or behavioural difficulties than those with asthma, diabetes or juvenile rheumatoid arthritis.[7–9]

The study described in this chapter considers children and families' experience of epilepsy and their attitude to stigma. Children's health beliefs both reflect and modify those of their families.[10 11] They influence coping strategies and adaptation to illness.[12] The notion that families may generate perceived stigma was advanced by Scambler and Hopkins, who challenged the view that stigma originates in a hostile public.[13] They suggested that "felt" stigma could predominate, and sometimes even predate "enacted" stigma as people avoid situations that could expose them to discrimination.[14] The term "stigma coaches" was later coined for those people, often parents, who encourage such secrecy.[15]

The narratives depicted here document the views of a group of children and families on why epilepsy is so distressing. They explore influences on the children's perceptions and contrast them with those of their parents and siblings.

Methods

The narratives are based upon interviews carried out in North London during 1997. Eighteen families on the paediatric epilepsy register of one hospital were invited to participate. Children with physical or severe learning difficulties were not contacted in order to focus on epilepsy specifically, nor, for practical reasons, were families who spoke little English. Six families consented, comprising six children with epilepsy, six mothers, three fathers and three older siblings. The two girls and four boys were aged between 8 and 12 and had been diagnosed 1–4 years previously. One child had developed seizures after meningitis but the others had an unknown cause. Half the children had absences and half generalised seizures. Families were from a range of socioeconomic groups. One family consisted of a single parent and child, the others two parents and siblings. The sample included Afro-Caribbean and white families but none from other ethnic communities.

The children were invited to talk freely about their epilepsy and to draw a picture of what epilepsy meant to them. The interviews were conducted by HW in the family home and lasted from 45 minutes to 2 hours. They were open ended, semi-structured and audiotaped with permission. Drawings were used, as a form of triangulation, to clarify and supplement their spoken stories. Parents and older siblings were interviewed individually and sometimes, in addition, as a family group. Interviews were analysed using the principles of grounded theory,[16] in which the raw data themselves form the basis for the analytical framework. Themes and constructs were developed by the author and refined after discussion with colleagues. All names of participants have been changed.

Results

Impact of epilepsy

These informants and their families felt that epilepsy had fundamentally altered their lives. A number of themes were apparent in the verbal narratives and the drawings:

Before the diagnosis – confusion and fear

Some children had experienced symptoms for some time before epilepsy was diagnosed. Absence seizures can be invisible even when attacks are occurring. This had led to delays in recognition and difficulty comprehending it. In some cases this had led to prolonged distress and educational difficulties. Children had been criticised for inattention or clumsiness and parents perplexed by obscure symptoms.

> He kept dropping drinks and I used to get so frustrated with him. And then when I was having a conversation with him but it was actually eye contact, when I noticed his eyes roll ... He had an EEG done which was really helpful at least we could see what was going on.
>
> *Ricky's mother*

Epilepsy as a strange and frightening happening

The initial shock of epilepsy made a powerful impact on these children. Their words and pictures vividly depict their incomprehension of epilepsy as a phenomenon. It is described as "weird", "strange", or "scary", and beyond their control.

> I was in my bed and it happened and I was sleeping and I didn't even know it had happened. I woke up and I am thinking "Mum, Dad why are you in here?" They go "You've had a fit and we have to get down the hospital quickly" and I am thinking "What?" It is like they haven't told me something, they are keeping something a secret and you don't know what

it is till they tell you. It feels weird, it feels like summat is really horrible.

Ricky

Being different

The unaccustomed sensations and emotions engender an intangible sense of difference both from their previous self and from others. The epilepsy, "it", has changed them.

> I call it absences. Well, it's like somebody's just turned out the light switch and everything has just stopped and sometimes I call them blackouts because everything just sort of turns off and I don't actually realise when I am having them until afterwards. It feels strange. Sort of, it's hard to describe because when I have them I don't actually know that I'm having them because it's just sort of switched off. ... I was writing something on the blackboard once like my teacher asked me to and I suddenly stopped and everybody started asking "Harriet Harriet", and I just wasn't there. ... It worried me at first because I didn't know what was happening and my teachers thought I was just day dreaming and it was sort of difficult to understand.

Harriet

The altered child

The children's perplexity is echoed by parents who describe an irrevocable and inexplicable change. Their child is no longer familiar. Known characteristics are perceived to have been replaced by new, strange ones. They also looked for explanations to understand and regain some control. They need to find meaning for their loss and guilt.

> ... and then he's gone and he's really gone. ... He didn't know who I was or anything. It was very strange. It's as though he wasn't really mine, you know, he was a complete stranger to me, even though he was my child. It was like I thought he was mad.

Darrell's mother

Explanatory models of epilepsy

Why me? Why my child?

Both children and parents indicated that they had been told by doctors that epilepsy often occurs for "no reason". But the search for a specific cause was apparent in their explanations. The nature and cause of epilepsy was sometimes confused with emotional stress and mental illness, and some informants were worried that it might cause behavioural or intellectual difficulties. This anxiety increased their sense of anomaly and isolation.

> It's not anybody's fault, they can get it for any reason, it just comes on. Then, you could be born with it. I may have had trouble coming out from my mum but I don't think that was the case. I think I caught a virus on the brain, I think that was it, that. There is loads of reasons. If you can't tell, you can't say, you ain't going to find out.... .
>
> *Jason*

> I suppose it would be different to other illnesses obviously but I don't know much about mental illness.
>
> *Katie's brother*

> They don't know there has been no obvious reason for it. I blame myself for it, maybe, I don't know. I smoked when I was pregnant, not many, but I think maybe if I hadn't have then he wouldn't, you know, just something. And I think if he hadn't run into the doorframe that day, if I'd been a bit quicker. If I'd done things differently when he was a baby perhaps he wouldn't. And when you see him and you can't help and think what have I done so wrong that makes him, to make him be that miserable, you know.
>
> *Ricky's mother*

An external agent

Bewildering changes within themselves were frequently attributed to an impetus from outside. Their pictures illustrate this. In Figure 7.1, the child wonders how he came to be recovering on the bed. Figure 7.2, by a child asked to "draw a picture about your epilepsy" shows an analogy with a light going out – someone else controls the switch.

> I was frightened. I'd just lost my father. I think Darrell was very very close to my Dad. Maybe it was there for a long time and it needed something to trigger it. He couldn't understand. He took in more than what I thought and it just kicked off something in his brain. I've come to terms with it. I don't blame God, some people they blame God, it's one thing I don't blame. It's one of those things.
>
> *Darrell's mother*

Living with epilepsy

A cross to bear

One of the most striking aspects of the children's stories is their perception of the continuous ordeal of having epilepsy. They are

59

constantly aware of its effect on their school life, holidays, friends, and family. The effort they exert to adapt to epilepsy and integrate it into their lives is significant and sustained. Their narratives reveal the complexity and responsibility the illness creates, and how it impacts on all aspects of their lives. Figure 7.3, the child under a thundercloud, sums up the emotions of all the informants.

> – Do you think about it all the time, or just sometimes?
> – All the time.
> – Do you? What do you think when you think about it?
> – Sad. I wish I didn't have it.

Katie

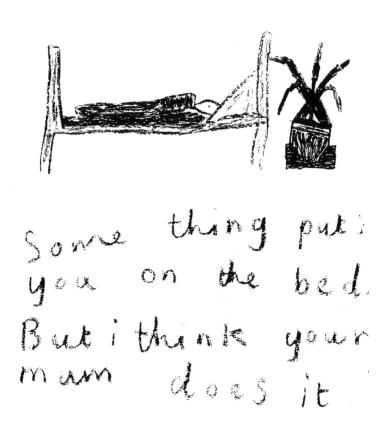

Figure 7.1 (Drawn by Patrick) After the seizure he's totally lost, he doesn't know who he is, where he is.

Patrick's mother

I might grow out of it. I wish I'd never had it.

Patrick

Yes, I still wish it would go away 'cause I could be like this forever and I don't want to be like that! It is hard. I'll just see how can I get through it and if I can I'll probably be the luckiest person on the Earth ... I want to get through it. It's like when you have a problem you can't sort it out and you have made it worse and you are thinking oh God, what's happening here? It feels horrible ... And that is my wish, just to get rid of it ... you've just got to get through it and then if you can't get through it, you can't get through it.

Ricky

[my friends] sort of didn't understand what was happening and I had to make them understand which was very hard. I tried to make them see that one, I wasn't contagious and two,

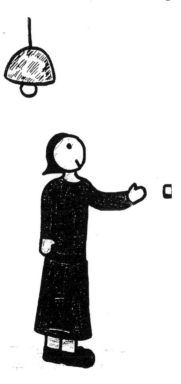

Figure 7.2   Well, it's like somebody's just turned out the light switch and everything has just stopped. It feels strange ... you say "this isn't me"

*Harrie*t

61

that I was going to be all right. Some of my friends went away with other people because they sort of got a bit frightened. It was hard for the first two or three months and then they sort of realised that nothing was sort of changing apart from my little absences ... I want to be my normal self again. I want to be able to not have to keep remembering to take my pill in the morning and evening. In the beginning I felt very very helpless ... I feel my normal self most of the time, it's just sometimes the thought of having to take medicine every day, just because this illness can get me down slightly.

Harriet

Medication – essential but constraining

Few children take regular medication, and the informants in this study perceived the need to take tablets as an unwanted responsibility that was both stressful and restrictive. Nevertheless, they understood the importance of not missing even a single dose.

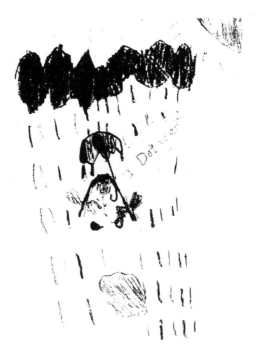

Figure 7.3   I wish I didn't have it
Katie

I've got to go away for a week [with the school] but the hardest part I think I will be going through is taking the tablets, maybe having too much fun, forgetting about them. ... So that's the chance I have got to take for myself. Don't forget them! Maybe it is hard work yeah but still it is probably the point of taking them. Or I will be ill forever.

Ricky

Because when I was seven, it brang me back, half my learning had gone 'cause of my brain so I had to build it back up again. You see I am only just getting to learn. I have to take them you see and I have to take them every day and if I stop taking them or if I forget, then I'll have one, I'll have a fit. And these are very important to me.

Jason

A "normal" life?

Once families got over the initial shock of the diagnosis, they tried to make life as normal as possible. Parents were anxious that epilepsy should not define their child but be just one facet of their character. Many said that epilepsy should not be what distinguishes the child from their siblings or peers. Parents perceived a difficulty in maintaining this attitude in the face of uncertainty and anxiety. The path between protection and overprotectiveness was often difficult to tread.

I don't tend to stand in the bathroom with him, I kind of pop up pretending to tidy up his bedroom and things so that gives him a bit of privacy – not overly protective but just ...

Ricky's mother

Keeping a balance was a particular challenge for parents when instilling discipline. They felt it important to be fair to all their children. They were sometimes uncertain whether misbehaviour or inattention should be attributed to epilepsy or medication. Again it was felt necessary to assess each situation and make a decision on the spot. They were aware that other adults may not be able to make the same judgments about their child.

He gets very angry and het up, I mean he is very stubborn but again he might just be like that. Or is it the fits?

Patrick's mother

63

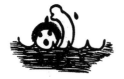 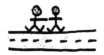

Figure 7.4   I'd like it to go away, 'cause I want to be my normal self again. I want to be able not to have to take my pill in the morning and evening. In the beginning I had to sort of be watched because the medicine didn't work straight away and so I had to be watched while crossing the road. In the pool I had to always have someone around me.

Harriet

> I think probably I can say I am softer on him than I would be. At the back of my mind I am always thinking "oh yeah he can't help the way he is". And I do think, even more when he is being really naughty, at the back of my mind I think to myself "is it this that's behind it?".
>
> *Ricky's mother*

The children themselves wanted to be treated as normal, neither cosseted nor ridiculed. They were young enough to accept some restrictions as a part of childhood. Figure 7.4 emphasises that swimming or crossing the road is safe if you take the medication. Despite a determined effort, however, they were always aware of restrictions attributable to their epilepsy.

> I am not allowed over the stream because of my fits. Because they say, if summat happens there and I could slip in and drown. I reckon that is a good point. I am not allowed to go past the corner shop by myself or with a friend ... The only thing I want is just get through and then go back to my normal life – I am a normal kid like everyone else.
>
> *Ricky*

The informants' siblings were also keen to play down the distinctions.

> I don't think she wants people coming round her and either giving her loads of attention or cold shouldering her because of what she's got.
>
> *Harriet's sister*

Invisibility and unpredictability

Unlike some other chronic illnesses, epilepsy is "invisible", but becomes apparent in unpredictable and dramatic ways. Parents recognised that, on the one hand, this allowed the children to present themselves as "normal" if fits were controlled, but also generated some uncertainty and apprehension. Because it is unseen, epilepsy becomes harder to understand and more frightening.

> It is difficult because he is perfectly normal and then all of a sudden he is like a light switch, just turn so and that's, it. ... Well at first, kids are kids, they didn't know what it was, you know they were a bit frightened, naturally, they're children. I try to explain to the other mothers the best I can but it's all, you know, "but he looks quite healthy".
>
> *Darrell's mother*

To tell or not to tell?

A misunderstood illness

Epilepsy was thought to be unseen and misunderstood not just by the child's immediate contacts but by society in general. The infrequent portrayals of the condition on television were viewed as negative and misleading. Difficulties envisaging the illness were felt to exacerbate misunderstanding, fear and discrimination. Some wondered if more obvious disabilities provoked greater understanding.

> Nearly every family now has got a child that has got asthma. With epilepsy it's just, it's so, "they are brain damaged", do you know what I mean? Obviously it is better for him that it can't be seen, he is not labelled as soon as he's seen ... but I am sure if someone is looking on an application form and it said, like, "epilepsy", people's first thought is "oh no, I don't want him having a fit in front of me" and someone in a wheelchair they'd know, at least they could, what's wrong with them. They're not going to have a fit in front of them are they?
>
> *Ricky's mother*

> They [other children] said I've got "Mad Boy Disease" ... My teachers don't know nothing about fits.
>
> *Patrick*

The invisibility of epilepsy requires the family to decide when to disclose the diagnosis. Whilst allowing them some control of the release of information, it also placed an added burden on the child and the family. None of the parents interviewed actively promoted secrecy; on the contrary, they encouraged honesty and self respect. However, they were also aware that such an approach might at times jeopardise their privacy or the child's social opportunities.

> I can't keep my feelings in I just let it out. I tell most people, not everyone, most people like know about it. I just like people to treat him normal, no different, you know, not contagious. I mean fair enough if you've never seen a fit then it would be frightening, but if I am around I can sort of tell them that I'm in control I know what's going on, don't worry.
>
> *Darrell's mother*

Another circumstance when parents thought disclosure important was to prepare others for the shock of witnessing a fit. Sometimes, however, they consciously withheld such warnings to prevent embarrassment or discrimination. Again there were ambiguities and families weighed and balanced each situation individually.

Fighting the stigma

A further consideration in the decision to divulge information was the desire to improve the public visibility of epilepsy and fight to reduce its stigma.

> [Katie's grandmother] said "I'm not telling anyone". I said, "Look, why not? I will, if you don't. There's no disgrace in it. She hasn't got to be locked up or in straitjacket. She is perfectly OK she is all right and I am not going to hide her away". I have no problem with people knowing. I'd rather them know, I really would, because then allowances will be made and I think allowances do have to be made.
>
> *Katie's mother*

> People should talk about it and should get it out in the open and then maybe our children will grow up not being ashamed of it or their children. It is a bit like asthma used to be with people, like "Oh God keep away from that child" whereas now everyone knows about it. I really hope that one day it will be the same for epilepsy, everyone will know and no-one will be judged for having it.
>
> *Ricky's mother*

A private burden

The children's attitude to publicity about their epilepsy was markedly different from their parents'. The fear of embarrassment or disgrace was overwhelming. They all described their reluctance to discuss it beyond the family and experiences of being teased or ostracised. Their "difference", the nature of the illness and the associations with madness that still pervade the playgrounds had all contributed. Even those children who, like their parents, said they should be open found it hard. They carefully selected one or two individuals to trust with their secret, sometimes using this as a sign of friendship. They expressed the firmly held view that the decision to disclose the diagnosis should be their own. Ironically, with adults they were more wary of over-protection.

> No-one knows I got fits except for my teacher. I haven't told them but they might know. Maybe my mum told them, maybe she has told their mums. They like, say things. Maybe they think it is a joke and all that, a laugh, but it isn't to me. I want to keep it as my secret. I know I should let them know. They know I have got asthma but they don't know I've got that. They don't know about my fits. ... I won't tell my best friend, I won't tell any of my friends I have got 'em. I know I should but it's just I don't. It's just, it feels as if it has got to be my secret, no-ones else's. ... I taked my choice that I didn't want to tell them.

> *Ricky*

> It's kind of personal like, kind of within the family like.

> *Katie's brother*

> I don't personally go around to everybody shouting "I've got epilepsy" ... It's sort of, it's private and when your friends see you having an absence then they'll understand but if you go sometimes to a parent they'll start sort of fussing all over you and it makes you feel very insecure and you feel very alone. So I try to avoid sort of saying "I've got epilepsy, will you be careful with me?"

> *Harriet*

Discussion

These narratives, albeit from a small and probably skewed sample of informants, provide a powerful impression of the profound impact of the condition on the life of the child and the family. The themes of incomprehension, sadness, and disempowerment were evident in all the interviews. The child has changed, their body is no longer reliable or understood. These families incorporated the changes but it required sustained effort to prevent epilepsy from dominating or restricting the child's independence and growth.

The families saw themselves as constantly trying to balance security and confidence against restriction and anxiety. The children want, and are strongly encouraged by their parents, to live a "normal" life, but still need special understanding and precautions. They carry the weight of secrecy, decision-making, difference, and loss of control. Even in supportive families such as these, it is a constant burden.

A further difficulty is the decision to disclose the diagnosis. This involves complex and flexible assessments of diverse variables. Even these young children worry about who to trust. They are vulnerable to unexpected embarrassment or harm; the risks of secrecy are balanced against the risks of disclosure. The fact that other previously stigmatised illnesses are now publicly discussed and understood makes it all the more frustrating that this one is not.

Perceived stigma developed in these children without overt parental encouragement of secrecy. Their unease was increased by the public invisibility of epilepsy which makes it difficult for others to envisage. Within their social context, a child's self esteem also depends upon an awareness of identity.[17] These children felt their body was no longer familiar. The continuity of their identity was interrupted and the intangible sense of difference intensified. Their stories suggest that felt stigma may be influenced not only by societal and parental beliefs but also by a feeling of difference and personal insecurity.

The children perceived epilepsy as an intrusion from outside. The metaphor is particularly powerful because of the symbolic association in our society of the brain with self and personality.[18] Furthermore the boundaries of self and the environment become indistinct so the child is unsure what is the illness and what is self. For a child at this stage of development, still mostly "concrete" in their thinking, it is a bewildering concept.[19] Their anxiety is increased by their belief that no-one else can appreciate what they feel. The hidden, unpredictable aspect of epilepsy has associations with shame or guilt. Its constant presence, even when invisible, means the child cannot recognise when they are safe. Such a combination of disempowerment and guilt may have long-term psychological implications. We should listen and understand when they "wish it would go away".

Acknowledgments

We wish to thank all the children and their families for telling their stories, and Dr Andrew Lloyd-Evans, Consultant Paediatrician, Royal Free Hospital NHS Trust, for all his help.

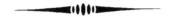

1 Kurtz Z, Tookey P, Ross E. Epilepsy in young people: 23 year follow up of the British national child development study. *Br Med J* 1998; **316**: 339–42.
2 Jacoby A. Epilepsy and the Quality of Everyday Life. *Soc Sci Med* 1992; **34**: 657–66.
3 Chaplin JE, Lasso RY, Shorvon SD, Floyd M. National General Practice study of epilepsy: the social and psychological effects of a recent diagnosis of epilepsy. *Br Med J* 1992; **304**: 1416–18.
4 Ridsdale L, Robins D, Fitzgerald A, Jeffery S, McGee L. Epilepsy in General Practice: patients' psychological symptoms and their perception of stigma. *Br J Gen Pract* 1996; **46**: 365–6.
5 Jacoby A. Felt versus enacted stigma: a concept revisited. *Soc Sci Med* 1994; **38**: 269–74.
6 Scambler G, Hopkins A. Generating a model of epileptic stigma: the role of qualitative analysis. *Soc Sci Med* 1990; **30**: 1187–94.
7 Austin JK, Smith MS, Risinger M, McNelis AM. Childhood epilepsy and asthma: comparison of quality of life. *Epilepsia* 1994; **35**: 608–15.
8 Hoare P, Mann H. Self esteem and behavioural adjustment in children with epilepsy and children with diabetes. *J Psychosom Res* 1994; **38**: 859–69.
9 Ferrari M, Matthews WS, Barabas G. The family and the child with epilepsy. *Fam Proc* 1983; Mar: 22 (1): 53–9.
10 Brett EM. "It isn't epilepsy is it, Doctor?" *Br Med J* 1990; **300**: 1604–5.
11 Bradford R. In: Bradford R. *Children, families and chronic disease. Psychological models and methods of care.* London: Routeledge, 1997.
12 Fitzpatrick R. In: Fitzpatrick R, Newman S, Thompson J, Hinton J and Scambler G. *The Experience of Illness* London: Tavistock Publications, 1984.
13 Goffman E. Stigma. Notes on the Management of Spoiled Identity. Harmondsworth, Middlesex: Penguin Books, 1968.
14 Scambler G, Hopkins A. Being epileptic: coming to terms with stigma. *Sociol Health Illness* 1986; **8**: 26–43.
15 Schneider J, Conrad P. In the closet with illness: epilepsy, stigma potential and information control. *Soc Prob* 1980; **28**: 32–44.
16 Glaser BG, Strauss A. *The discovery of grounded theory.* New York: Walter de Gruyter, 1967.
17 Barnes P. In: Barnes P. *The Personal, Social and Emotional Development of Children.* Oxford: Blackwell, 1995.
18 Helman C. *Culture, Health and Illness*, 3rd edition. London: Butterworth Heinemann, 1994.
19 Piaget J. *Judgment and Reasoning in the Child.* New York: Harcourt Brace Jovanovich, 1976 (first published 1928).

The conker tree

Trisha Greenhalgh

I was more resentful than usual about being on call. Earlier, the children had waved me off to Saturday surgery and asked if I would be back for lunch. We'll go to Hampstead Heath and look for conkers, they had said, hopefully.

But it was now 1.30 pm and there seemed little chance of any daylight hours with the family. I had seen the usual stream of worried well and one genuine emergency. Sulkily, I chewed on a dry cheese sandwich in the car on my way to visit an 83-year-old lady who had developed a dense paralysis the day before.

Unusually for a right sided stroke, it had not affected her speech. This was fortunate, for she had a long story to tell. She had been born in this house and married at 19 to the boy next door. After a childless 64-year marriage in which they enjoyed good health and their own company, he had awoken recently with chest pain and died in her arms, minutes before the ambulance arrived.

She had never entered a hospital until a fortnight ago. Now, with the winter bed crisis already apparent in some places, I had no alternative but to pack her off to the same casualty department when, days previously, a newly qualified house officer had performed the perfunctory routine on her husband's corpse before politely taking his leave to deal with the living.

A friend fussed about, gathering clothes and toiletries, while I scribbled a referral letter. Then we fell silent, waiting for the ambulance. My professional task was complete, but there were no pressing calls and I felt compelled to wait and see her off.

"Do you want to see his wreath, doctor? Look out of the window: it's in the garden."

The floral tribute in the shape of her late husband's name lay wilting on the patio table. The garden was beautifully tended, with autumn colours in the flower beds and a neat, lush lawn. In the middle was a magnificent horse chestnut tree, and the grass was thickly strewn with the best conkers I had ever seen.

She was quick to notice the direction of my gaze.

"Have you got children, doctor?"

"Yes. Two little boys."

"Well, go and get some conkers. Dot, give the doctor that plastic bag. I can wrap my nightie round the sponge bag. We planted that tree when I was pregnant 50 years ago, but I lost it on Christmas day and I never caught on again."

I let myself out of the back door. It was like running into virgin snow. I gathered armfuls of shiny fat conkers until the bag was full to bursting. The ambulance arrived as I was putting it in the boot of my car.

"Do come back and help yourself, doctor. You can climb over the back gate. They're no use to me now, you know."

That evening, my boys gleefully divided the loot between them and I feasted on a moment she had dreamed of but never known. Their thank-you letters were returned later by the hospital: R.I.P.

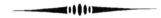

Narrative in medicine

8 Pain narratives

Sir Richard Bayliss

Pain is one of the most common symptoms proffered by patients, not infrequently being their main and often their only complaint. The narrative comes pouring out as, in a haphazard way, they "spill the beans" in their own words without structured thought. Not only must the physician hear what is said but with a trained ear he or she must *listen* to the exact words that the patient uses and the sequence in which they are uttered. In addition patients use another method of communication – body language – of which they are usually quite unconscious. The recipient of the narrative must keep both ears and eyes open to receive these two equally important complementary narratives.

Even if the patient's narrative was recorded verbatim by a stenographer, it would lose much of its significance to a third party, and there would be no account of the body language involved. In the clinical context the doctor has not only to hear and see the verbal and visual presentations but must also record the essence of them – a few words in the GP's notes or a longer account by the house-physician on the ward. To the tidy-minded professional the temptation to interrupt the patient in order to clarify ambiguities or to obtain more details must be steadfastly resisted until the patient has finished. Histories must be received, not taken.

The exact words and the sequence in which they are used often provide an invaluable clue to the diagnosis and, surprisingly, many patients say exactly the opposite to what they really mean.

Mrs Trumper, aged 45, a clerical officer with Westminster City Council, was ushered into the out-patient consulting room. We shook hands and she sat down. She smiled and her opening words were, "I'm happily married but I have the most terrible headaches." I stopped her because I wanted to see how many of the four medical students sitting with me had heard what she had said. I handed each of them a slip of paper and asked them to write down the patient's exact words – precisely that she'd said. Three recorded that Mrs Trumper had "severe headaches", and only one that she was "happily married and had severe headaches". None, apparently, had observed the smile on her face. "You may have heard but

75

only one of you has listened," I said to the students quietly (and confidentially) "Why has this patient had to tell us that she is happily married? What possible reason is there for her telling us that before she mentions her headaches? There must be a reason, probably a quite unconscious one. I suspect that we'll find that Mrs Trumper is *unhappily* married." And so it turned out.

"If after receiving a history and asking supplementary questions you haven't got a pretty good idea of what the diagnosis is, you probably never will" may be an old-fashioned truism. It is, I submit, as true today as it ever was, despite a computer program jogging your memory about some cause of abdominal pain that you have long forgotten about, such as porphyria. Nevertheless birds on the lawn are usually sparrows or wrens and seldom ostriches. When in a fix we are all guilty of sending off blood to the laboratory for tests that are less sensitive and less specific than a well recorded history.

The 25-year-old woman lay on a trolley in A&E; her eyes screwed up; her face contorted in pain. "It started in the back of my head – suddenly – about an hour ago. Something seemed to go pop inside. The pain spread down the back of my neck and then all over my head. It's terrible." She clasped her head with her hands. The patient's body language, her description of the pain and the something that went pop inside her head gave the diagnosis. It took only seconds to show she had photophobia and nuchal rigidity as a consequence of her subarachnoid haemorrhage.

In 1937 a notice appeared on the board in the School of Pathology at Cambridge University announcing that the Regius Professor of Physic would give a lecture at 12 noon. Who on earth was the Regius Professor and what did he do? And what exactly was 'Physic'?

Sir John Ryle, previously an honorary consultant physician at Guy's Hospital in, of course, the pre-NHS days, was the new Regius Professor. Despite a busy private practice, he had done much research on gastro-intestinal disorders, being particularly interested in the relationship between gastric secretion, gastric acidity and peptic ulcer. Hence Ryle's tube. Aware of the schism that in those days existed between pre-clinical and clinical medical education, he gave a series of lectures to provide stepping stones to bridge that unnatural divide.

Tall, lean, with greying hair and immaculately dressed without over-doing it, he spoke clearly without a note or a slide for 50 minutes, keeping his audience spell-bound. His topic was The

Clinical Study of Pain.[1] When confronted with a patient complaining of pain, there were eleven features that needed elucidating – not in every patient, of course, but in those in whom the cause of the pain or the diagnosis was difficult or uncertain. He warned us not to interrupt the patient as s/he delivered the narrative but we could make brief notes as a reminder to question the patient later about those aspects that needed clarifying.

Six years later, in 1943, as the medical registrar at St Thomas's Hospital (there was only one in those days) one of my tasks was to take Medical Sorting Room every morning from 10 am until 12 noon. To this clinic patients with medical disorders were referred, without any appointment being required, by general practitioners from far and wide. The Casualty Officers would also refer to it medical patients that walked in off the street.

This was before the epidemic of coronary artery disease. The hospital had one ECG machine, the size of a bed and about as unwieldy to manoeuvre. There was no technician. If an ECG was requested by one of the consultant physicians, the medical registrar took it, and developed and printed the photographic plate. Only Leads I, II, III and a single chest lead were recorded.

The Clinic was held in a large windowless white-tiled room, reminiscent of a huge Victorian lavatory. Bare wooden benches with hard backs were arranged in neat rows on the terrazzo floor. The medical registrar sat at the far end of the room, perched on a high chair with a narrow sloping desk in front of him and the patient far below on an ordinary wooden chair – an arrangement hardly conducive to a close doctor–patient relationship. Intimate exchanges were inhibited by the tiled walls which ricocheted the narrative into the ears of those waiting silently on the crowded benches.

"Next please."

The patient left his seat on the front bench and walked quietly to the desk. He handed me a doctor's visiting card on which was written: "Mr Boreham, aged 55. Please see and advise". I noted with little surprise that the general practitioner lived in Woking. Many patients who lived in the south-east commuted to Waterloo Station and found it more convenient to be seen in the Metropolis.

"Do please sit down, Mr Boreham. How can I help you? What d'you do in life?"

"I'm a senior civil servant at the Home Office. I keep getting a pain ... a sort of tightness ... here in my chest". He clenched his right hand and placed it over the centre of his sternum. "I live in Woking, you see, but work at the Home Office and come to London by train every day. I get this pain in the mornings after breakfast as I walk to the station. I know it sounds odd but the pain comes on when I get to about the fourth or fifth lamp-post down the road from our house. I have to stop and if anybody saw me they might think it rather peculiar", he smiled, "so I pretend I'm looking at the scenery or at one of our neighbours' gardens. After the tightness has gone, I go on to the station. There's quite a steep incline up to the platform. If I'm a bit late and hear the train coming, I have to hurry and the pain comes on again just about the time I open the carriage door."

I learnt that the pain lasted about 3 or 4 minutes, and had first started 3 months ago. The patient never got the pain going home in the evening. Once or twice it had occurred after he'd had lunch at his club in St James's and was walking up the slight incline to Piccadilly, particularly on a cold or windy day.

"It's deep inside somewhere. Not sharp but a pressure, almost a crushing feeling like a vice. At the same time I may have a curious feeling here in my jaw and sometimes, hurrying up to the platform at the station, there's a heaviness in my left arm too. Here ..." He ran his right index finger down the inner side of his left arm as far as the elbow.

Twenty minutes later, after asking more questions and having found nothing abnormal when I examined Mr Boreham in one of the little cubicles behind a partition wall, I perched myself at the desk again. I dabbed my rubber stamp on its ink-pad and pressed it on a page of the notes. Then I filled in the answers to John Ryle's 11 questions (Table 8.1).

Table 8.1   The case of Mr Boreham – Ryle's checklist

Situation	Central retrosternal.
Radiation	To jaw and down left inner arm to elbow.
Localisation	Deep in the chest.
Character	Tightness, crushing, vice-like. Clenches fist.
Severity	Definite and severe.
Duration	For 3 months; lasts 3–4 minutes.
Frequency	Every a.m. walking to station.
Relieving	Standing still.
Aggravating	Inclines, hurrying, cold or windy days, after food.
Special times	Walking to station in am or up St James's.
Associated symptoms	None. No shortness of breath.

The value of Ryle's checklist is, of course, much greater in patients in whom the diagnosis is not as obvious as it was in this patient but I reproduce it here to show how succinctly the historical data can be recorded. Ryle's list can be used for the elucidation of pain anywhere – in the chest, the abdomen, the back, the limbs, the face and the head – but the narrative may need some clarification before its essential features are entered in Ryle's list.

Situation. Patients have an extraordinary concept of where the abdomen is – anywhere between the middle of the chest and the symphysis pubis. When undressed, have the patient show you precisely where the pain is. Gastric or duodenal ulcer pain is usually felt in the epigastrium but if a duodenal ulcer is eroding into the pancreas it may also cause pain in the back; colonic pain may be felt in the lower abdomen or be more accurately located along its anatomical course; renal pain usually in the loin or flank.

Radiation. This can be helpful, even diagnostic. Ureteric pain is often referred to the ipsilateral testis in men and the labia in women; upper right quadrant abdominal pathology, such as a subphrenic abscess, to the tip of the right shoulder; chronic cholecystitis to the scapular or interscapular area; pancreatic pain to the back. The pain of appendicitis or of ovarian pathology may be referred to the ipsilateral lumbo-sacral area. Pain from salpingitis or a tubal pregnancy may be referred to the front of the thigh.

Localisation. Beware of the roving hand! A flat hand moved in circles over the whole abdomen seldom indicates organic disease. In peptic ulcer the site of the pain is usually indicated in the epigastrium with the tips of two fingers.

Character. The adjectives used vary with the educational and cultural background of the patient. "Crushing" and "vice-like" are often used to describe the pain of angina or of myocardial infarction which is seldom, if ever, "knife-like". Peptic ulcers induce a "gnawing" or a "dull toothache-like" pain. Gall-bladder pain is often "bursting". Small intestinal pain caused by infection or obstruction is griping, rhythmical and intermittent. Biliary or renal colic may be colicky but often increases in an unremitting crescendo. "Burning" pain or "heart-burn" in the upper epigastrium or lower chest, relieved by burping, is usually due to an hiatus hernia or oesophageal reflux. Burning pain elsewhere in the abdomen is seldom caused by organic disease.

Severity is difficult to assess. I used to think that "agony" was an exaggeration probably indicative of non-organic disease but no

79

longer. Today "agony" is used in many cultures for describing labour pains; it cannot be discounted. Severity is also often reflected in the narrative of body language. Facial expression and hand gestures are important. Sweating, pallor, tachycardia and shock are physiological body language. Severe pain is not amenable to distraction.

Duration of the pain may provide a vital clue to the diagnosis. Anginal pain seldom lasts more than a few minutes because the patient stops doing whatever provokes it. The pain of myocardial infarction or biliary or renal colic may last for hours until relief is brought with potent analgesia. Peptic ulcer pain is episodic and seldom lasts more than an hour, until milk or food is taken in the case of a duodenal ulcer or the stomach has emptied in the patient with a gastric ulcer. The pain of a gastric carcinoma is less influenced by eating and is often unremitting.

Relieving and Aggravating factors are complementary, the two sides of the same coin, and may provide important clues to the pathology, but often you may have to ask the right questions. Patients with a duodenal ulcer have "hunger" pains, especially in the night, which are relieved by a glass of milk or an alkaline medicament. Gastric ulcer sufferers often note the repeated relationship between their pain and meals. Pressure applied to the abdomen may ease intestinal colic or spasm but not inflammatory diseases. Pain that occurs only on exercise or exertion is nearly always ischaemic in origin. Angina may occur in many sites, not just the heart or the legs but in the arms, masseter muscle and elsewhere. Being jolted in a car or on a horse may precipitate renal or biliary colic or induce colonic spasm.

Special times help to clarify aggravating and relieving factors.

Steve was an old patient who for 30 years had come for an annual check-up. At his initial consultation he'd said, "I've checked – we're the same age, so you're the right man to keep an eye on me over the years. We'll grow old together." And over the years we did. He worked in Lloyds and lived well, a keen golfer with a handicap of three. He was, typically, not averse to consultations at the 19th hole! He was about 65 when on an annual visit he told me he'd got trouble with his right hip. He'd consulted an osteopath friend at the golf club but without benefit. He'd also consulted a physical medicine doctor, another club member, but he'd done no good either. So what hope had I of reaching a diagnosis other than osteoarthritis of the right hip? In due course I was able to complete Ryle's list.

The "hip pain" was in fact felt in the right buttock. It did not radiate. It only came on after Steve had walked for a certain distance, particularly up an incline leading to his farm, and it went as soon as he stopped walking. On examination the hip and back movements were relatively full and painless. Certainly the X-rays he brought with him showed some degenerative changes and osteophytes as one would expect in a man of his age, but it needed an aortogram to confirm that the intermittent claudication in the right buttock was caused by severe atherosclerotic narrowing of the right common iliac artery. And how come that the two experts had not noted the reduced pulsation in Steve's right femoral artery? Perhaps it was a recent development. The vascular surgeon did him well.

Some patients complain of pain that is not characteristic of anything. You may have to put them "on hold" and start all over again next time they come to see you, but by using Ryle's schema you may be able to decide whether the pain is of organic origin or not. Functional pain often has weird radiation that defies the anatomy, and the physiology, of the nervous system. In such patients the words and body language used to describe the pain are often bizarre, being either over-dramatic or accompanied with apparent indifference.

Mrs Bruford, the middle-aged wife of an accountant, looked downcast as she sat beside the desk in my consulting room. The corners of her mouth curled down, suggesting unhappiness or discontent; her clothes were fashionable but shabby; her hand-bag was scuffed and her shoes surprisingly unpolished. Her problem was pain which, on analysis, started in her left lower chest anteriorly. It would come on suddenly as a sharp "fizzy" feeling, she said. It would shoot suddenly anywhere – down her left leg or up the left side of her neck; sometimes she felt it "fizzing all the way down my right arm." The pain lasted only a matter of seconds. It worried her because her mother had had the same pain and she had died – but in a car accident it emerged. It did not take long to learn that Mrs Bruford was indeed unhappy – with her husband and with her two teenage children. As I listened to her I began to feel depressed. Clinical depression is a surprisingly contagious condition and doctors readily "catch" it from their patients. Further questioning revealed that Mrs Bruford fell asleep quickly enough but always woke at 2 am and seldom got off again until shortly before it was time for her to get up. The diagnosis was not in doubt.

In such patients it is sometimes surprisingly easy but in others quite impossible to lead them gently to the realisation that pain may occur without any physical disease or structural abnormality being present but it may take a lot of time.

Bernard Lown, an outstanding American physician, in his book, *The Lost Art of Healing*,[2] is concerned about the current failure in the United States to take the kind of history that so often unmasks the diagnosis before a hand is laid on the patient. In the United Kingdom the same often applies, not because we are not taught how to receive a proper history but because we do not have the time. You need time to listen to a pain narrative and the patient needs time to give it you. The requirement to see more patients in less and less time is neither in the patients' best interests nor in the doctor's because it reduces his intellectual satisfaction in his work. Therein lies the rub.

Incidentally John Ryle left Guy's Hospital at the age of 46 in 1935 to take the less arduous post of Regius Professor of Physic at Cambridge because he had developed angina. In 1943 he moved to Oxford to be their first Professor of Social Medicine. He died in 1950 at the age of 61, having lived with his angina for 16 years.

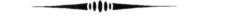

1 Ryle JA. *The Natural History of Disease*, 2nd edition. Oxford: Oxford University Press, 1948, pp. 36–51.
2 Lown, B. *The Lost Art of Healing*. Boston: Houghton Mifflin, 1997.

9 Following the story: continuity of care in general practice

Iona Heath

> ... the lives of great artists and poets and writers are not, after all, so extraordinary by comparison with everyone else. Once known in any detail and any scope, every life is something extraordinary, full of particular drama and tension and surprise, often containing unimagined degrees of suffering or heroism, and invariably touching extreme moments of triumph and despair, though frequently unexpressed. The difference lies in the extent to which one is eventually recorded, and the other is eventually forgotten.[1]

Stories are the basic tool and the great reward of general practice, with the capacity to enrich the lives and the experience of both patient and doctor.[2] Stories give an account of events, people, emotions and feelings that extends over time, and this longitudinal dimension is fundamental to the long-term relationship between doctor and patient that underpins general practice. For many patients, the general practice record, whatever its limitations, is the only sustained written record of their lives. The existence of this concrete documentation of their suffering, coping and endurance gives tangible form to the general practitioner's role as witness to the patient's unfolding life story.[3]

Shared stories

Stories are told throughout medicine, but only general practice offers the possibility of doctors and patients sharing their stories over more than half a lifetime. My own experience suggests that a young doctor starting in a practice forms special relationships with certain cohorts of patients. The most obvious of these are with patients of the same gender and approximately the same age. The doctor and these patients progress through life together, having children, dealing with the failing health of older relatives and coming to terms with their own ageing, all at much the same time. Cultural and historical events, both local and national, are more powerfully held in common because they impinge on doctor and patient at roughly the same point in each individual lifecourse.[4] In the words of Elwyn and Gwyn (Chapter 17), doctor and patient share both historical and 'event' time. They exchange stories over many years – stories that vary from those reporting the comforting minutiae of daily life to those that grapple with the need to keep going in the face of overwhelming personal disaster.

I have noticed that other particular relationships are formed with those patients who are approximately the same age as the doctor's parents and those of the same generation as the doctor's children. The doctor shares the ageing of older patients at the same time as being part of his/her own parents' struggle to retain their dignity and enthusiasm for life in the face of deteriorating health and the loneliness that must follow the loss of family and friends. With the younger cohort, the doctor's expertise and confidence is consistently heightened while dealing with those particular children who are roughly the same age as his/her own. And when the doctor's own children are indulging in the ritualistic risk-taking of adolescence, it can seem much easier to make at least some sort of contact with those young patients whose struggle for independence and identity is leaving them with a sense of being frighteningly out of control.

These generational relationships are particularly strong but the vast majority of general practice patients share stories with their doctor on numerous occasions over long periods of time. These shared stories form powerful bonds which can actively enable trust and effective care. However they can also become rigid and codified, and lead to dangerous presuppositions and complacency that can blind the doctor to significant changes in the patient's state of mind or body.[5] Doctors need always to strive to see and hear the patient afresh however strong the bond of shared history, perhaps by following the example of Isaiah Berlin.[6]

> What interests me is what is wrong with the ideas in which I believe – why it is right to modify or abandon them.

Stories of illness

The patient comes to the doctor to tell the story of his or her illness; to give an account of when she first became aware of things being not quite right with her body or her mind, of how it all seemed to begin, and how it developed to the point when she felt that she must seek the attention of her doctor. The story may include details of who else she has told and from whom else she has sought advice, of what she and others may think may have caused the problem to arise at this particular point in time. However, the evidence suggests that the patient's whole story is seldom heard. On average, the doctor interrupts after only 18 seconds of the patient's narrative.[7] Yet, if the patient is allowed to proceed, the full story lasts, on average, only 28.6 seconds,[8] which seems not much to ask of the listener.[9] Indeed, a lot may be gained by encouraging the story-teller to develop the narrative to include as much as possible of the rich psycho-social context in which the symptoms are embedded.

Almost all patients can be encouraged to venture a theory of causation attributing the development of symptoms perhaps to a fall or other minor accident, or to a particularly stressful situation either at home or at work.[10] Often these attributions will prove entirely correct, but sometimes they are used to conceal the fear, and sometimes the reality, of the random misfortune of developing a malignancy or other life-threatening disease. Not many patients openly express their fears of incurable or fatal disease but such fears lurk unexpressed in most consultations and if they remain unacknowledged may continue to fester, closing down communication between doctor and patient.

Stories of disease

> Illness is what the patient has on their way to see the doctor and disease is what they have on the way home.

> *Anon*

Having listened to the patient's account of his/her symptoms, the doctor seeks those parts of the narrative that fit the stories of disease, the patterns that medical science has defined in an attempt to make sense of the suffering caused by illness, and to find relief or cure.

> Doctors travel back and forth across the bridge, taking the patient's story of illness to be informed by medicine's abstract knowledge and then to be interpreted and returned to the patient as a presumptive diagnosis retold in the form of a case history.[11]

85

It is essential that the patient's story is not distorted and coerced to fit the patterns of science. The common illness symptoms including headache, tiredness, abdominal pain and many others, can all be caused as much by stress and unhappiness, as by more or less serious disease. Scientific medicine offers much benefit but also carries great dangers as the frightening prevalence of iatrogenic disease testifies. If illness caused by unhappiness, anger, loneliness or grief is misinterpreted as being due to disease, the patient will be exposed to the dangers of scientific medicine without the possibility of benefit. Society may also incur the very considerable costs of high tech medicine.[12]

As Marshall Marinker demonstrates in Chapter 11, the symptoms and suffering caused by unhappiness are no less real because they do not fit the disease template of scientific medicine. Doctors need always to remember that what the patient feels is the reality on which they must base their practice. The taxonomy of diseases represents the nearest science has got to nature, but it remains a theoretical construct. It is the theory that should be discounted when the patient's symptoms refuse to fit, not the patient's account of the reality of their experience.[13] Only by continuing to listen attentively to our patient's stories of illness will we increase the accuracy and the usefulness of medicine's stories of disease.

Stories of endurance

Once the technical transactions of medicine are complete, general practitioner and patient still have to come to terms with the debility, pain and fear that comes with illness and disease. Scientific medicine can sometimes cure, but often can provide no more than amelioration of symptoms. Many doctors sense failure in the absence of a cure and retreat from their patients when their need for support and solidarity is greatest. When there is no cure and no scientific explanation for the arbitrariness of suffering, it is necessary to construct a narrative of endurance and survival. This task is central to the relationship of general practice, in which the general practitioner and patient may be left to find a way forward together after the specialists who investigate and attempt cure have dropped away. Patients coping with the pain, humiliation and loneliness of, for example, chronic mental illness or coping as a survivor of domestic violence, need to construct a story through which they can rediscover a sense of self worth and of dignity.

These narratives of endurance can be seen woven through human history, and the patterns of these narratives date back to the earliest myths that define the cultures of the world. The story may be one of courageous survival in the face of terrible ill-luck, or of the tragic victim of human carelessness or malice, or of fierce struggle against apparent destiny. Through such stories, patients are able to make some sort of sense of what has happened to them, and to take comfort from the stories of others, in fiction, film or journalism, who appear to have suffered in a similar way.

Stories can accommodate suffering and give a meaning to experience, but if the story is allowed to become fixed, the patient can become trapped within the narrative. Too rigid a story closes off choices and opportunities to move beyond traumatic experiences. Sometimes the doctor can offer the patient a different story which could enable them to see a way forward. The patient may have settled for the role of tragic victim and yet be capable of a shift to that of courageous survivor which can offer much more scope for renewed self determination, dignity and self respect. The classical exemplar for this liberating progression is Sophocles' Philoctetes.[14]

Literacy: medical, physical, emotional, cultural

If the full potential of the patient's story is to be realised, the doctor (and perhaps particularly the general practitioner) needs to be willing to listen, to hear and to be literate at many different levels. Medical literacy ensures that where the patient has a disease for which medicine offers effective treatment then the pattern of the patient's symptoms will be recognised and appropriate action taken. Physical literacy[15] makes use of the doctor's subjective awareness of his or her own body, combined with his or her objective knowledge of the body as a biological specimen. This combination underpins the empathic interpretation of the patient's symptoms which lies at the root of diagnosis. Emotional literacy[16] allows the doctor to acknowledge and witness the patient's suffering and pain, and to help in the struggle to find a way forward. Cultural literacy enriches the search for meaning[17] with examples of the way others have made healing sense of the same sorts of hurt and pain.

The education of doctors gives them knowledge of how the health of individuals and populations could be improved. This gives doctors a responsibility to retain a vision of how the health of each individual could be improved. Depending on the particular circumstances, this vision will include social, psychological, physical, economic, nutritional and environmental elements. The vision can be seen as a different story for the patient, which should never be imposed but which can be made available to the patient so that they have a share in the knowledge of how their health could be improved and can make informed choices.

Poets have a similar responsibility to provide an alternative vision and no-one writes more eloquently of this responsibility than Seamus Heaney:

> it is essential that the vision of reality which poetry offers should be transformative, more than just a print-out of the given circumstances of its time and place.

He understands an imagined alternative view as offering not only the possibility of change but also an aid to endurance and survival.[18]

The power of poetry lies in its evocation of all that is common to human experience enabling individuals to feel less alone. John Berger touches on the same area in his discussion of two dimensions of time:

> Man is unique insofar as he constitutes two events. The event of his biological organism – and the event of his consciousness. Thus in man two times coexist, corresponding with these two events. The time during which he is conceived, grows, matures, ages, dies. And the time of his consciousness.[19]

Wisdom acquired through exploration of the time of consciousness can be used to change the story of a life within biological time.

Stories that bridge cultures

One of the great privileges of working in general practice in inner city London is the cultural richness of the stories that patients bring. These stories originate from cultures across the world and from a huge breadth of social settings. Nonetheless the extraordinary persistence of common themes and preoccupations emphasises, again and again, our shared humanity.[20] Every story contains a new truth with the capacity to extend the understanding of the doctor.

Yet the attempt to tell stories across cultural boundaries often founders on linguistic barriers. Clearly, the transactions of general practice are severely impoverished in those consultations where patient and doctor do not even share a common language and when they bring very different cultural frameworks to the consultation. On some occasions only medical literacy is left; it is seldom equal to the task and both doctor and patient are aware of the inadequacy.[21] As Vieda Skultans shows in Chapter 22, deliberate and sustained efforts are needed to overcome these barriers. Practitioners need to learn to work constructively with bilingual interpreters and health advocates in ways which enable patients to feel that their story has been both told and heard.

The end of the story

> Few of the tragedies at life's end are as rending to the clinician as that of the frail elderly patient who has no one to tell the life story to. Indeed, becoming a surrogate for those who should be present to listen may be one of the practitioner's finest roles in the care of the aged.[22]

The processes of dying and death bring the patient's story to a close. Knowledge of, and sensitivity to, the patient's narrative helps the doctor to see the end of the patient's life as a fitting culmination of that life rather than the failure which death becomes within the more usual transactions of scientific medicine.[23] Through seeking to understand and value the story, the doctor seeks to understand when the threat of death is untimely and when it ceases to be so.

A few years ago, one of my patients suffered a heart attack. She was a woman of 92 who I remember having carefully instructed me on the benefits of keeping cut flowers in fizzy lemonade rather than water. She was admitted to the coronary care unit of one of our local teaching hospitals and given intravenous streptokinase. She made a gradual recovery and was discharged home 10 days later. I went to visit a day or two afterwards to find her in a state of shock which seemed to be mostly to do with how little her aspirations for her life had been understood. She had been a widow for many years, she was severely disabled by advanced chronic obstructive airways disease and she had, by then, lost almost all the friends of her own generation. She wanted to be cared for in a way which preserved her dignity but she was no longer concerned with survival for its own sake. She viewed the treatment she had been given as self evidently impressive but, in her case, invasive and inappropriate. She was very shaken by her experience of the best of scientific medicine and she died quietly in her sleep 2 weeks later.

Time and space for story-telling

Stories can only be told when people have time to talk and time to listen and to hear. The richer the narrative the more time is needed. The magnificent advantage of general practice as a mode of clinical care is its longitudinal dimension and the opportunities this gives both doctor and patients to develop and respond to complex narratives in relatively short instalments but over a sustained period of time. However if the instalments are too short, the stories can become constrained and thereby less effective. John Howie and his team in Edinburgh[24] have demonstrated that with longer consultations patients are more likely to respond affirmatively to the following six questions:

As a result of your visit to the doctor today, do you feel you are:

- able to cope with life?
- able to understand your illness?
- able to cope with your illness?
- able to keep yourself healthy?
- confident about your health?
- able to help yourself?

Howie describes these as giving a measure of enablement, the ability of the patient to cope with their illness experience within the particular context of their own life story. The achievement of enablement correlates with the length of the consultation, providing further evidence that general practice consultations should average no less than 10 minutes in length.

Teaching, research, health promotion, patient care that was previously undertaken in hospital, and care in the community, are all important, but all take time. Rising time pressures diminish the capacity of general practice with potentially disastrous results:

> Unless consultations are understood as the points of production of critically important decisions which determine all other consumptions, the cost-effectiveness of the entire NHS will fall in terms of net health gain, even if it improves in terms of reduced waiting times or raised outputs of technical procedures. The quality of consultations must in large part

depend on freedom from time pressures, without perverse incentives to save time by ill-considered somatisation, prescription or referral, and with protected time in which to develop patients' capacities as producers rather than consumers.[25]

If the additional tasks are to be quite properly accommodated, more general practitioners will be needed in a medical workforce which is already inadequate.[26] Without increased capacity, general practitioners may no longer have time to seek an understanding of the patient's narrative, to the detriment of both parties to every consultation.

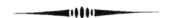

1 Holmes R. *Footsteps: adventures of a romantic biographer.* London: Hodder and Stoughton, 1985.
2 Borkan JM, Miller WL, Reis S. Medicine as storytelling. *Fam Pract* 1992; **9**(2): 127–9.
3 Berger J, Mohr J. *A fortunate man:* the story of a country doctor. Harmondsworth, Middlesex: Penguin Books, 1967.
4 Backett K, Davidson C. Lifecourse and lifestyle: the social and cultural location of health behaviours. *Soc Sci Med* 1995; **40**: 629–38.
5 Gulbrandsen P, Hjortdahl P, Fugelli P. General practitioners' knowledge of their patients' psychosocial problems: multipractice questionnaire survey. *Br Med J*; **314**: 1014–18.
6 Quoted in Currie C. Old fools, rogues, lovers, and sages. *Br Med J* 1997; **315**: 1102.
7 Beckman HB, Frankel RM. The effect of physician behaviour on the collection of data. *Ann Int Med* 1984; **101**: 692–6.
8 Svab I, Katic M. Let the patients speak. *Fam Pract* 1991; **8**: 182–3.
9 Coulehan JL. Who is a poor historian? *J Am Med Assoc* 1984; **252**: 221.
10 Malterud K. Women's undefined disorders – a challenge for clinical communication. *Fam Pract* 1992; **9**(3): 299–303.
11 Jones AH. Literature and medicine: narrative ethics. *Lancet* 1997; **349**: 1243–6.
12 Barsky AJ, Borus JF. Somatization and medicalization in the era of managed care. *J Am Med Assoc* 1995; **274**: 1931–4.
13 Rudebeck CE. Humanism in medicine. Benevolence or realism? *Scand J Prim Health Care* 1992; **10**: 161–2.
14 Heaney S. *The Cure at Troy.* Derry: Field Day, 1990.
15 Rudebeck CE. General practice and the dialogue of clinical practice: on symptoms, symptom presentations and bodily empathy. *Scand J Prim Health Care* Suppl 1/1992.
16 Adam S. Presentation at the launch of the Chief Medical Officer's Annual Report for 1996. Royal College of Physicians, 29th November 1997.
17 Midgeley M. *Science as salvation: a modern myth and its meaning.* London: Routledge, 1992.
18 Heaney S. *The redress of poetry.* London: Faber and Faber, 1995.
19 Berger J. *And our faces, my heart, brief as photos.* London: Writers and Readers, 1984.

20 Lambert H, Sevak L. Is "cultural difference" a useful concept? In: Kelleher D, Hillier S. *Researching Cultural Differences in Health.* London: Routledge, 1996, pp. 124–59.
21 Yee L. *Breaking Barriers: towards culturally competent general practice.* London: Royal College of General Practitioners, 1997.
22 Kleinman A. *The illness narratives: suffering, healing and the human condition.* New York: Basic Books, 1988.
23 Towell D. Revaluing the NHS: empowering ourselves to shape a health care system for the 21st century. *Policy Politics* 1996; **24**(3): 287–97.
24 Howie JGR, Heaney DJ, Maxwell M. *Measuring Quality in General Practice, Occasional Paper 75.* London: Royal College of General Practitioners, 1997.
25 Hart JT. *Feasible socialism: the National Health Service, past, present and future.* London: Socialist Health Association, 1994.
26 Medical Workforce Standing Advisory Committee (MWSAC – The Campbell Committee). *Planning the medical workforce*, 2nd report. London: Department of Health, 1995.

10 Narrative and mental health in primary care

John Launer

Introduction

Throughout this book, different writers point towards a tension that runs through medicine in the late 20th century. It is the tension between the complex narrative which the patient brings into the consulting room and an apparent understanding by the doctor of what is *really* going on, as formulated in a diagnosis or an idea about pathology. Which is a truer account of reality: the patient's or the doctor's? Can both be true? If so, how?

In much of the medical world these questions are still being asked in whispers, but in mental health they are becoming a roar. There are many reasons for this. First, there is the influence of sociology and ethnography which have identified psychiatry as peculiarly culture-bound among the medical specialities.[1-4] Then there is the cultural position of psychiatry itself, in an uncomfortable no-man's land between conventional medical science and a search for meaning which extends into political and religious domains.[5] Another factor may be the jumble of confusing and contradictory languages which different mental health professionals use to describe their observations. In a Babel of explanatory models which often appear to disqualify each other, or simply to be a way of asserting the therapist's power, the patient's own story may gain in authority and occasionally appear saner than the professional's.[6 7]

However, the most important reason for the so-called "narrative turn"[8] within the world of mental health may be a different one altogether: namely, that psychiatry is the only area of specialist medicine where talking and listening are explicitly understood to be therapeutic. Historically, the one idea from Freud which has now conquered all the various fragmented and cacophonous schools of mental health care is that of the "talking cure".[9] (The phrase, tellingly, was invented not by Freud but by his patient, Bertha Pappenheim.)

In a recent book on narrative in family therapy,[10] Papadopoulos and Byng-Hall point to a major change in our understanding of what the "talking cure" actually involves. They describe how clinicians from many different therapeutic schools are now moving away from the search for any normative explanation of someone's problems, and towards the search for an appropriate *new story* for each patient. They argue that this change has its origins in modern and "post-modern" intellectual movements, including cybernetics[11 12] and structuralism.[13]

Other contemporary mental health professionals have given similar accounts of this change. For example, the influential American therapists Anderson and Goolishian argue for the need to abandon "paradigmatic" models that test the patient's experience against some pre-determined view of normality.[14] They propose an approach which acknowledges the client as expert and which is prepared to facilitate any possible account of reality, provided that it makes sense in the client's own eyes. In the same vein, Burck refers to selfhood as something to be "produced" rather than "discovered".[15] What all these ideas have in common is that the conversation between clinician and client can no longer be regarded as a tool for seeking out hidden truths. Instead, it is a means of creating previously unformulated ones.

The reader who encounters such ideas for the first time, whether or not a mental health clinician, often reacts with some incredulity. Is there any place in this anarchic, post-modern universe for facts or professional expertise? Are we not in danger of alienating our psychiatric patients, who surely come to us looking for certainties rather than a regress of deconstructions? This chapter is not the place to give an account of the intense debates that have raged around these questions nor of the positions that have been taken on them, from the extremes of revisionist brain theories ("mental illness comes from brain biochemistry alone") to the equally fundamentalist extreme of radical constructivism ("even birth and death are only the inventions of language").[16 17] However, it is important to note that many mental health professionals have now taken on board a dilemma which has been exposed at the heart of our work: *how do we hold on to our own theories and beliefs, while allowing the patient's story its full opportunity to evolve, even if it does so in directions we might neither expect nor wish?*[18–20]

The narrative therapist in practice

Rather than giving a theoretical response to this question, I want to present some clinical cases where there are apparent mental health problems, together with some commentary on the challenges presented by taking a narrative approach to them.

In my professional life I am mainly a GP but I have a special interest in opportunities for mental health work in general practice.[21] I am a trained family therapist and also involved in teaching at the Tavistock Clinic.[22] In my clinical GP work I am aware of narrative in three of its aspects:

- in its familiar role in taking a traditional medical history;[23]
- in its counselling aspect, as something which needs to be listened to, allowing patients to give coherence to their own history;[24-26]
- as a therapeutic stance which involves questioning the patient in a way that explores *new meaning which may make a difference to the patient.*[27]

It is this last aspect which interests me most and which I want to address in the cases that follow.

To some extent the cases are random: they were the first three patients booked to see me in one particular morning surgery not too long ago. I have altered biographical details to conceal identities. The commentaries are an attempt to recapture some of the mental processes by which I try to sustain a narrative-based therapeutic stance while continuing to remain aware of the pressure (and often the need) to take other stances in the consultation, including paternalistic or "expert" ones.

Case one

Helen is in her mid-seventies. She sees me every month for high blood pressure. However, we usually deal with the blood pressure very quickly because we have other important things to talk about. Helen was widowed about 10 years ago and immediately offered to share her home with an elder sister. Tragically, the elder sister began to develop Alzheimer's disease. For the years that followed, Helen was torn between her sense of responsibility and an awareness that her sister's needs could break her own health. She

95

battled to keep the situation afloat, and sometimes we fought together for resources against an inadequate welfare system.

Eventually, 2 years ago, Helen's sister went into a nursing home; and recently, she died. She had become mute, doubly incontinent and unable to recognise anyone, although Helen always visited her daily. So you will understand that our consultations are not spent just measuring blood pressure. We talk about Helen's grief, and also her relief. She still has some unresolved guilt about putting her sister in a home: who wouldn't? In addition she has a terrible sense of waste: why did her sister have to end her life in this apparently meaningless way? Why has Helen had to spend her own widowhood having to toil away desperately, so that she now faces her own old age exhausted and quite depressed?

Commentary

I have intentionally described Helen's case in the manner of a doctor telling the story to colleagues, not as one might present a psychiatric case history in a journal. So it is already in a "narrative" rather than "paradigmatic" form. It ranges longitudinally over a period of years rather than just giving a snapshot of one moment. It involves not just the patient but also the system which surrounds her: the family, and agencies of the state. It appears to move indiscriminately between the domain of mind and that of the body. I am present in the stories myself as agent. It is my own narrative of Helen's narrative; she might tell it differently. It is the stuff of most general practice, framed predominantly in biographical rather than pathological terms.[28]

As a GP working in the real world, one question I have to struggle with is this: is Helen "suffering from depression"? How do I hold up the predetermined, quasi-scientific template of psychiatric diagnosis against my personal reading of Helen's story? GPs, like all clinicians, are under pressure to give a diagnosis: from our training, from managers, from the journals which bombard us, and from institutions like the Royal Colleges which are exhorting us to "Defeat Depression". Yet a diagnosis is actually no more than a linguistic construct, often designed for the needs of one profession but serving others' needs awkwardly or not at all.[29] Used thoughtfully, a diagnosis may be a helpful convention designed to help the physician in order to help the patient. Used without thought, it can become a tool for fending off the doctor's anxiety.

It may also generate inattention to any parts of the patient's story that might create cognitive dissonance for the doctor.

One solution to this challenge is to see my main work as being not just to listen to Helen, nor just to formulate diagnoses, but to ask questions which explore a better story: the story of Helen not as a declining person who has failed and thus become a psychiatric case but of a conscientious sister who did her best when faced with an atrocious dilemma. I am, in other words, committed to exploring the "subjugated discourse",[30] or the story of the "underdog".[31] I want to emphasise that this does not preclude offering Helen the diagnosis of reactive depression, or even suggesting anti-depressants. However, if I do these things I want to do so collaboratively, trying to find out if such suggestions fit her own view of her story. If she chooses in response to cede authority to me ("Do you think I should take pills, doctor?"), that is also part of the narrative that I have to take into account.[32]

Case two

Rustem is Iranian, in his fifties, and recently out of prison where he served five years of a sentence for assault. While he was in prison his wife started divorce proceedings. But in spite of this, they are currently living together as he has nowhere else to go. I look after all the family, so I was involved when Rustem's mother died from cancer 4 years back and I had to arrange for him to have compassionate leave from the prison to see her on her death bed. He visited her in handcuffs. I have also seen a lot of Rustem's wife and sons. They have talked about the shame and the economic consequences of having a breadwinner who is a criminal and a convict. Incidentally, Rustem's wife is a seamstress and each Christmas she makes and brings me a pair of trousers.

Now Rustem has come out of prison as a heroin addict. I see him fortnightly to prescribe methadone. However, Rustem also has major medical problems, including quite severe rheumatoid arthritis, and I am trying to sort these out too. It is hard because Rustem comes in with enormous pressure of speech and I cannot manage to clarify one problem before he moves onto the next. His English is not very good and I speak no Farsi at all. In spite of my sympathy with his wife, I believe he has been deeply traumatised psychologically by his stay in prison and is depressed. I do not know how he will deal with divorce and presumably eviction.

Commentary

Rustem's case makes me ask myself the question (half ironically): is his mental health problem *serious*? On the one hand, I might say that it was not terribly serious, because there is no obvious psychosis nor even any "biological" features of depression. On the other hand, Rustem may be a worrying candidate for suicide, given his age, his impending divorce, his unemployment, his history of violence and his drug habit. So how are we to judge the seriousness of the stories we hear and take part in?

Seen in terms of the complex, poignant narratives in which many doctors participate daily, it is hard to avoid being sceptical about the way the mental health world community now divides up its workload, into "serious pathology" and the so-called "worried well". This trivialises much of our daily work, or reduces it to a troubling two-dimensionality. Also, it may run the risk of being a self-fulfilling prophecy. If you compartmentalise your narrative so that the categories of the psychotic and violent are cut off from their family and social context, you may be amplifying exactly the problems you are trying to help. (For example, once we have given people the label of schizophrenia, however justified, we may stop trying to have normal conversations with them about their lives, and thus contribute further to a process of marginalisation.) Of course, we do need to make some distinctions about risk and complexity and difficulty in the stories we hear. However, the more of the patient's story we listen to, the less discrete and static these distinctions may appear.

As a GP, I believe I have to do two things. I have to acknowledge that I am sometimes dealing with genuine danger – to myself, to my patients, and to their relations – and that in the real world I can get into serious trouble if I ignore it. But I also have a responsibility not to pathologise people by seeing their stories in only one way.[33][34]

Case three

I was originally asked to see 3-year-old Sheryl and her mother by one of our health visitors. The mother is sometimes a lone parent, sometimes not. Her relationship with Sheryl's father is an on–off, violent one. Sheryl herself has major behaviour problems: she hits her mother and also the other children in her school. She shouts and screams and bites. Mother and daughter have had some involvement with social services and the local child guidance clinic but nothing seems to help. They fail to engage with help, or it appears to work for a very brief time and then they quickly disengage. Each time, the mother returns to my surgery with Sheryl to ask if there is any other approach she can try. A year ago I arranged for a placement at the local family centre, where I hoped they would be able to do some structured family work. However, Sheryl's mother had to work during the day so this too failed as an intervention.

Recently, against the wishes of all the previous agencies involved, she has requested a referral to an expert on childhood hyperactivity disorder in the hope that Sheryl's problem can be solved by medication.

Commentary

My main difficulty here concerns the idea of treatment, or solutions. Like every GP, and every other mental health worker, I am under enormous pressure to deliver cures, preferably at great speed. Yet my own understanding of Sheryl's story is that it does not invite quick solutions. It has evolved out of a matrix of genetics, family and social influences, together with moral choices and fate. The mother's view is that there is an instant cure just around the corner. My own belief is that my long-term role will probably be as the constant figure among a shifting community of professional carers, able to tolerate this family's cycle of unrealistic hopes and subsequent disappointments. Whose narrative is "right", mine or hers?

One way I try to respond to this question is by refusing to be wedded to either narrative – either the one created by her impulsive optimism, or my own rather fatalistic view. So I am prepared to make referrals such as the one she is requesting, even against my own beliefs or instincts. At the same time, I have to allow myself to realise that there may well be social, economic and other forces which make any hopes for a different story rather fanciful. Others, including possibly the hyperactivity expert, may disagree.

Conclusions

The commentaries I have given on these cases draw attention to the problems posed by an attempt to reframe our encounters with mental health problems in terms of stories. The story-telling approach may collide rather violently with concepts imported from positivist, "objective" viewpoints. Narratives are not necessarily about categorisation; they may be about lack of boundaries. Clinicians who stand at the intersection between the world of stories and the world of categorisation, between the hermeneutic role[35] and the World Health Organisation's International Classification of Diseases (ICD-10), may well feel that theirs is an impossible position.

One possible route leading away from this dilemma may be offered by the field of thought known as social constructionism.[36–38] According to pure social constructionism, all types of knowledge – including professional knowledge – can be seen as mere stories which we negotiate among ourselves as agreed versions of reality, often as a means of exerting power. However, a less fundamentalist version of constructionism accepts that some stories may approximate more or less to testable, scientific reality, although they can never exactly reach it. What characterises this view, therefore, is not a rejection of medical activity in the name of hermeneutic purity, but an acceptance of the shared roles of patient and doctor in *exploring, creating and testing the efficacy of new stories*.[39]

Seen in this light, the medical consultation can be understood as an opportunity for a dialogue between different stories: the biographical one brought by the patient, and the professional one brought by the doctor. The doctor's contributions may come in all sorts of forms, including interpretations about the family origins of a problem. However, they may also come in the form of a biomedical story (for example, an account of the genetics and biochemistry of schizophrenia) or as a proposed action such as a drug treatment or referral. Indeed, if mind and body are seen as an interactive field, then all medical interventions – even psychopharmacology – can be seen as an agreed intervention into the patients' *storying* of themselves. The doctor's contribution to the story can thus be valued not as truth which has prior and superior validity to that of the patient, but only in so far as the patient finds the doctor's contributions to the plot useful.

———————◼◖◗◖◗◼———————

1 Lock M, Gordon D eds. *Biomedicine examined.* Dordrecht: Kluwer, 1988.
2 Hahn R, Gaines A. *Physicians of Western medicine.* Dordrecht: Reidel, 1985.
3 Kleinman A. *Patients and healers in the context of culture: an exploration of the borderland between anthropology, medicine and psychiatry.* Berkeley: University of California, 1980.

4 Lupton D. *Medicine as culture: illness, disease and the body in Western societies.* London: Sage, 1994.

5 Stevens A, Price J. *Evolutionary psychiatry.* London: Routledge, 1996.

6 Szasz T. *The manufacture of madness.* New York: Harper and Row, 1970.

7 Masson J. *Against therapy.* London: Collins, 1989.

8 Brown D, Nolan P, Crawford P, Lewis A. Interaction, language and the "narrative turn" in psychotherapy and psychiatry. *Soc Sci Med* 1996; **43**: 1569-1578.

9 Freud S. Five lectures on psychoanalysis. In: *The Standard Edition of the Complete Psychological Works of Sigmund Freud, Volume 11.* London: Hogarth Press, 1909.

10 Papadopoulos R, Byng-Hall J eds. *Multiple voices: narrative in systemic family psychotherapy.* London: Duckworth, 1997.

11 Bateson G. *Steps to an ecology of mind.* New York: Ballantine, 1972.

12 Keeney B. *The aesthetics of change.* New York: Guilford Press, 1983.

13 David R ed. *Lacan and narration: the psychoanalytic difference in narrative theory.* Baltimore: John Hopkins University Press, 1983.

14 Anderson H, Goolishian H. The client is the expert: a not knowing approach to therapy. In: McNamee S, Gergen K *Therapy and social construction.* London: Sage, 1992.

15 Burck C. Language and narrative: learning from bilingualism. In: Papadopoulos R, Byng-Hall J eds *Multiple voices: narrative in systemic family psychotherapy.* London: Duckworth, 1997.

16 Hoffman L. A reflexive stance for family therapy. In: McNamee S, Gergen K eds *Therapy and social construction.* London: Sage, 1992.

17 Parry A. A universe of stories. *Fam Proc* 1991; **30**: 37–54.

18 Frosh S. Post-modernism versus psychotherapy. *J Fam Ther* 1995; **17**: 175–90.

19 Pocock D. Searching for a better story: harnessing modern and post-modern positions in family therapy. *J Fam Ther* 1995; **17**: 149–73.

20 Orange D. *Emotional understanding: studies in psychoanalytic epistemology.* New York: Guilford Press, 1995.

21 Elder A. Psychotherapy in general practice. In: Maxwell H ed. *An outline of psychotherapy for trainee psychiatrists, medical students and practitioners*, 2nd edition. London: Whurr, 1993.

22 Launer J, Lindsey C. Training for systemic general practice: a new approach from the Tavistock Clinic. *Br J Gen Pract* 1997; **47**: 453–6.

23 Hunter K. *Doctors' stories.* Princeton: Princeton University Press, 1991.

24 Shapiro J. The use of narrative in the doctor–patient encounter. *Fam Sys Med* 1993; **11**: 47–53.

25 Cole-Kelly K. Illness stories and patient care in the family practice context. *Fam Med* 1992; **24**: 45–8.

26 Maine M, Caplan N, Cassidy J. Security in infancy, childhood and adulthood: a move to the level of representation. In: Bretherton I, Walters E. *Growing points of attachment theory and research.* Monograph of the Society of Research and General Development, Serial No. 209, Volume 50, Numbers 1–2. Chicago: University of Chicago Press, 1985.

27 Launer J. A social constructionist approach to family medicine. *Fam Sys Med* 1995; **13**: 379–89.

28 Gordon P, Plamping D. Primary Health Care. Its characteristics and potential. In: Gordon P, Hadley J eds. *Extending primary care.* Oxford: Radcliffe, 1996.

29 Armstrong D. Construct validity and GPs' perceptions of psychological problems. *Primary Care Psychiat* 1996; **2**: 119–22.

30 Flaskas C, Humphreys C. Theorising about power: intersecting the ideas of Foucault with the 'problem' of power in family therapy. *Fam Proc* 1993; **32**: 35–47.

31 Campbell D. The other side of the story: the clients' experience of therapy. In: Papadopoulos R, Byng-Hall J eds *Multiple voices: narrative in systemic family*

psychotherapy. London: Duckworth, 1997.

32 Launer J. "You're the doctor, doctor!": is social constructionism a helpful stance in general practice consultations? *J Fam Ther* 1986; **18**: 255–68.

33 White M. Negative explanation, restraint and double description: a template for family therapy. *Fam Proc* 1986; **25**: 169–84.

34 Cecchin G, Lane G, Ray W. *Irreverence: a strategy for therapists' survival.* London: Karnac, 1992.

35 Mendez C, Coddou F, Maturana H. The bringing forth of pathology. *Irish J Psychol* 1988; **9**: 144–72.

36 Hazzard A. Measuring outcome in counselling: a brief exploration of the issues. *Br J Gen Pract* 1995; **45**: 118–19.

37 McNamee S, Gergen K. *Therapy and social construction.* London: Sage, 1992.

38 Harré R. *The social construction of emotions.* Oxford: Blackwell, 1986.

39 Speed B. Reality exists O.K.? An argument against constructivism and social constructionism. *J Fam Ther* 1991; **13**: 395–409.

11 Sirens, stray dogs, and the narrative of Hilda Thomson

Marshall Marinker

In a monograph entitled *The Order of Things*,[1] Michel Foucault quotes a Chinese encyclopaedia in which animals are divided into the following categories: (a) belonging to the Emperor, (b) embalmed, (c) tame, (d) sucking pigs, (e) sirens, (f) fabulous, (g) stray dogs, (h) included in the present classification, (i) frenzied, (j) innumerable, (k) drawn with a very fine camelhair brush, (l) etcetera, (m) having just broken the water pitcher, (n) that from a long way off look like flies.

The day before I wrote this article I saw a patient, whom I will call Hilda Thomson, during a morning surgery at a village health centre. She was new to the district, having moved into the village about 3 months ago. She was in late middle age, a large, rather untidy woman with an angry looking face. It was clear that she did not have very high hopes of the consultation. She told me that she had increasingly severe pains in her arms and legs, and that these had been made infinitely worse by a visit to an osteopath in the city. Her only reason for visiting him, she said, was the signal failure of doctors to help her in the past.

Some years ago she had been diagnosed as suffering from rheumatoid arthritis. In support of this story she produced from a canvas bag some eight or nine bottles containing examples of most of the current remedies for this condition and, of course, by way of an hors d'oeuvre and a dessert, a selection of choice psychotropic drugs and a sleeping tablet. The pain had been made much worse by the move to the village. Three years ago, she and her husband had bought a grocery shop in the nearest town and had commuted about 30 miles from their previous home. A year ago her husband, Peter, who had previously taken a large part of the burden of the shop, had had a coronary thrombosis. Since then he had become a complete invalid, demanding constant attention, refusing to venture beyond the garden gate, and taking no part at all in the running of the business. She had been taking the sleeping tablets for 3 years, but habitually woke in the small hours of the morning. Three years ago blood tests had suggested the diagnosis of rheumatoid arthritis. Inspection of her joints now revealed little evidence of the disease, although her eyes filled with tears when I began to examine her. She told me that the Government was unfair to small shopkeepers and that nobody in society cared about the "little man".

The problem which is posed by the classification of animals in the Chinese encyclopaedia is similar to the problem posed by the events and perceptions of the consultation with Hilda Thomson. After all, what astonishes the reader of the Chinese encyclopaedia is not the elements of the taxonomy, but that mysterious schema which links them together. Foucault comments on "the stark impossibility of thinking *that*".[1] It is starkly impossible because we cannot imagine what the taxonomy was meant to accomplish. It is simply not recognizable. The only link that we can see between animals belonging to the Emperor, animals included in the present classification, and those drawn with a very fine camelhair brush, is that they appear together in the imagination of a long dead encyclopaedist.

What about the present imagination of the general practitioner who encounters Hilda Thomson? Consider his (or her) list: serological evidence of rheumatoid arthritis 8 years ago; the purchase of a grocery shop 3 years ago; the coronary thrombosis of the patient's husband; an angry face and voice; a shopping bag full of tablets which have not helped; tears of pain when the wrists and knee joints are palpated; and a belief that society does not care about the "little man". Just to utter the contents in the way that I have done is to invite Foucault's comment on "the stark impossibility of thinking *that*". Yet a habit of practice, if not yet a system of thought, encompasses both the results of the serological tests and the political complaint. It is not easy to say on which plane of the imagination these ideas meet. But the challenge of those who teach general practice is to offer a coherent taxonomy for ideas such as these so that they make sense to young students who will be encountering other Hilda Thomsons in their professional future.

The view from the hospital

As long ago as the 18th century, the Edinburgh Clinic was organized so that "those cases which seem most instructive" might be brought together. In tracing the birth of a modern teaching hospital to its roots in the 18th century, Michel Foucault in his *Naissance de la Clinique*[2] uses the word "clinic" with two meanings. It describes not only the teaching hospital, but also the medicine practised within it. The same word embraces both the location of the practice and the system of ideas which it houses. The clinic, in this sense, is no longer simply a meeting place between doctor and patient. It is a system of thought, a field of pathology, a language which articulates the human experience of being unwell. The development of a pathological nosology generated the language which we use to describe what we see and, at the same time, excluded from the discourse those parts of the encounter between the doctor and his patient with which the new language could not deal.

In the name of vocational relevance, it has been argued that the teaching of clinical medicine should shift dramatically from the study of patients with lobar pneumonia in the hospital to a study of patients with such conditions as acute bronchitis and acute tonsillitis at home, simply because the latter conditions are much more common than the former in our society. But it is important not to blur the argument. What cannot be asserted is that there are differences in the nature of diseases manifested in the hospital and diseases manifested in the patient's home. Only the distribution of morbidity will be different. The basic concepts of disease processes, the pace and sequence of events, the appearance of tissues, both to the naked eye and through the microscope, the notion of cause and our classification both of causes and effects are not materially different in the study of lobar pneumonia and acute tonsillitis, and they are unaffected by the location of these events.

Indeed, since the notion of a disease is essentially abstract – an ideal model, a template against which the more untidy experiences of individual doctors and their patients can be tested and observed – the clinical teacher could quite properly argue that extremes, however rare, are the best models for teaching.

No-one could suggest that an encounter with Hilda Thomson, who complains miserably of pains in her knees, a husband who abdicates his manhood, and a society which no longer cares for the "little man", is useful for learning about the pathogenesis, symptoms, physical signs, X-ray and laboratory characteristics, or natural history of the idea of rheumatoid arthritis; still less that the taxonomy of joint diseases will be best explicated by countless encounters with men and women who complain of an ache here or a pain there which can only be ascribed to a pathological event by the most strenuous exercise of the iatric imagination.

The *idea* of the disease is best taught on the best models available, and the best models available occur in the hospitals. This is a tautology. The *raison d'être* of the modern hospital is the discovery and manifestation of diseases and their management. By definition it is in the hospital that the best diseases – the most florid, the most spectacular, the most intriguing – will manifest themselves. Of course these same diseases occur outside the hospital also. But here they are disguised; they lurk beneath the surface of appearances and events, so much so that the anger in the patient's face may distract our gaze from the results of the serological test, or the overwhelming presence of the person, Hilda Thomson, may mask the *idea* of her rheumatoid arthritis.

A medicine of persons

There is a paradox which lies at the root of modern medicine. The science of persons – whether we are talking about pathology, human pharmacology, psychology, or sociology – is concerned to discover generalisable truths which are demonstrable not in individuals but in groups. The natural history and clinical findings of measles, mumps, cancer of the breast, or schizophrenia are true only of the ideas of these diseases. Clinical method is concerned to compare the reality of the unique individual with the model of the ideal disease. The degree of proximity between the reality and the ideal will determine the diagnosis and the confidence with which it is made.

The benefits of this clinical method have been enormous. It has made possible a scientific medical discourse about the individual and the same method has been followed in the behavioural sciences. But this discourse profoundly determines the way in which we look at ill health, the ill health which we are prepared to recognize and value, and the relationship within which the commerce between doctor and patient takes place.

Consider, for example, the extraordinary phenomenon of depression as a late 20th century diagnosis. In a review article on depression[3] the following were described as classical psychological changes: lowered mood; difficulty in thinking; loss of interest; delusional ideas; hallucination and depersonalization. The following were described as classical physical changes: sleep disorders; weight loss; constipation; reduced libido or sexual potency; and disturbances of menstrual function.

Contemporary psychiatry has invented a nosography of diseases modelled closely on diseases of tissues, organs, and chemistry. For the most part, this nosography refers to beliefs or fantasies which are acceptable only because they are consonant with modern biochemical explanations. Slowly but surely the patient is learning to present the human experience of unhappiness to his or her doctor in terms of depression. A different system in France teaches the patient the vocabulary of liver disease in the face of similar human experiences.

I would like to advance the argument that a medicine which regards the patient not only as an object but also as a subject continues to exist in general practice, even though it can be discerned only in the shadows cast by the towering edifice of the hospital. It persists precisely because the patient refuses to be ill according to the best precepts of modern medical education.

I do not want to give the impression that general practice disdains the concept of diseases. What I have been at pains to do is to point out those many untidy facts and perceptions which persist beyond the discourse of tissues, organs, and chemical reactions. In the case of Mrs Hilda Thomson, the discourse about tissues and organs brilliantly articulates the idea of rheumatoid arthritis and helps to explicate the remedies that we can offer. But these solid three-dimensional objects, like swollen deep-red synovial membranes or clots of blood, do not take us very far in understanding the relationship between Hilda and Peter Thomson, his heart attack, her arthritis, her anger with him for withdrawing from his commitments, the reasons for his retreat, her feelings that nobody, society, the Government, or perhaps simply the doctor, cares for the "little man".

This part of medicine, because it is outside the discourse of tissues and organs, hardly appears at all in the written tradition of modern medical science. However, it persists in the oral tradition of medicine, and in my day it persisted in the oral tradition of clinical teaching in the medical school. I think that it did so for two reasons. The first is that the medical school teacher of earlier generations was often still a generalist; but of equal importance was the fact that he was not an academic. Particularly in the English medical school, the tradition of academic departments is relatively recent.

What is the role of the academic clinician? What, in the language of Thomas Kuhn,[4] are the paradigms in which he or she works? The academic specialist's major task is to advance the knowledge of his subject, and to do so he thinks and works within the boundaries of scientific fashion within the paradigms of physiology and biochemistry. Of course these intentions are good and the results are enormously valuable to mankind. But the system of values which this way of working creates – the view of man (or woman) as an object not a subject and the belief that the clinical task is to distinguish the clear message of the disease from the interfering noise of the patient as a person – constitutes a threat to medical humanism.

Specialism, which we created because the burden of our knowledge became unbearable, subserves this dehumanising process. The threat is made more menacing still when, in both teaching and practice, the domain of the patient's feelings and emotional life is treated as though it too were a fragment of specialist medicine, to be dealt with by the psychiatrist.

The general practitioner is faced with a number of competing images of Hilda Thomson. Small joint pains with evidence of early thickening or deformity, and a positive serological test for rheumatoid some years ago, project one image. But there are clues, even in this short consultation, that there has been intense domestic bargaining for the role of sick person. There is evidence not only of inflamed synovial membranes, but also of inflamed resentments. The sleepless nights, the hint of sexual abstinence, at least since the coronary thrombosis a year ago, and the sense that medicine and osteopathy can provide no relief from the pain constitute fragments of a diagnosis which is largely missing from the written tradition of clinical medicine.

The problem of choice in medical diagnosis is akin to the problem of choice in art or poetry. Statements in art contain many truths which do not compete with one another in the way that scientific formulations compete. Of course the dispute between rheumatoid arthritis, tuberculous arthritis and gouty arthritis, must be resolved in the diagnosis of Hilda Thomson's painful wrist. But we do not need similarly to resolve the images of her anger towards her husband, her resentment of society, her sexual frustration, her rejection of medication, or her anxieties as a shopkeeper, in the same way. Nor do these images compete with the pathologies of her joints or of her husband's coronary arteries.

The sum of all these images constitutes the approximation of a truth about Hilda Thomson's problems.

It is these rich realities that lie behind the somewhat arid statement that general practitioners compose all their diagnoses simultaneously in physical, psychological, and social terms. I believe this concept to be central to the act of general practice.

Post script

This chapter was originally written in 1977.[5] I was intending then to hint at the challenges facing general practice as a newly formed academic discipline. I used the term 'general practice' as Foucault uses the term *'la clinique'* to describe at one and the same time a location of practice and also a philosophy of medicine. I would not want it to be thought that this philosophy of medicine which I value is always to be found in general practice and is never to be found among the other medical disciplines. This is simply not so. The virtue of general practice is that, by the very nature of its extended and untidy nosography, these aspects of medicine cannot be hidden either from the doctor or the student.

Earlier in this chapter, I asked, "On what plane of the imagination do the changes in Hilda Thomson's joints, the look of anger, her husband's interminable convalescence, and her complaint about society's lack of concern for the 'little man' meet?" It is not on the planes of pathology, sociology, or psychology, but on that plane of the imagination which embraces the concepts of whole-person medicine. This sort of medicine requires from the doctor not only a knowledge of the language and grammar of diseases, but also of human mythology, a mythology that reaches deep into the origins of the species, the ethnic group, and the society. Furthermore, it requires from the doctor an ability to handle the ambiguities and contradictions both of his patient's experience and his own responses. It is in this sense that these disparate and messy ideas constitute a holistic taxonomy of human health. The task of academic general practice remains now, as it was 20 years ago, to explore, create and apply such a taxonomy in the pursuit of the doctor's prime task – to come to an understanding with the patient about "what is wrong" and "what is to be done".

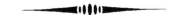

1 Foucault M. *The Order of Things*. London: Tavistock Publications, 1970.
2 Foucault M. *The Birth of the Clinic*. London: Tavistock Publications, 1973.
3 Parry-Jones WL. Depression. *Update* 1973; **6**: 491–6.
4 Kuhn T. *The Structure of Scientific Revolutions*. Chicago: University of Chicago Press, 1962.
5 Marinker M. The chameleon, the Judas goat and the cuckoo. *J Roy Coll Gen Pract* 1978; **28**: 199–206.

12 Narrative in surgery

James Owen Drife

Surgery has been called, by one of its leading practitioners, "a somewhat repulsive cruel craft, modestly modified by ... scientific principles".[1] Admittedly, this description referred to the era before Lister and it may be less apt nowadays after the introduction of anaesthesia and asepsis. Nevertheless, the business of surgeons is deliberately to wound and sometimes to mutilate their fellow human beings, and this sets them apart from other contributors to this book on narrative based medicine.

Contrary to popular belief, surgeons are no less cultured than doctors in other specialties. Most surgeons enjoy reading, seeing plays and listening to music. When I was a junior doctor, it was a consultant surgeon who told me that however hard I was studying I should always read a novel for half an hour before going to sleep. At the time I thought his advice revealed a frivolous approach to life but nowadays I relax in front of the television set before going to bed. Movies are the new narrative form of the 20th century and *Casablanca* on video is the grown-up's version of the child's familiar story.

This chapter, however, is not about the use of the narrative (in the form of literature or film) as an escape from surgery or as therapy for the stress of operating. Nor is it about the central place that surgical operations play within the illness narratives of patients,[2] though an analysis of this phenomenon could form a chapter in itself. Instead, I have focused on how the narrative dimension of illness and healing explored elsewhere in this book in relation to *medical* practice might relate to the very different discipline of surgery.

Barriers to "narrative based surgery"

A good case has been made for the fundamentally narrative based nature of the physician–patient relationship in both mental health (see Chapters 10 and 18) and primary care (see Chapters 9 and 11). The authors of these and other chapters in this book have taken as their starting point the notion that the clinical arts of caring and curing occur as an unfolding and negotiated story (see Chapter 1). It is not difficult to make a list of reasons why surgery sits less easily in such a narrative paradigm.

Actions, not words

Narrative depends mainly on words but surgery requires actions. The surgical specialties are distinguished from other branches of medicine by an over-riding demand for dexterity. This began in the pre-anaesthetic era when amputations had to be finished within a few minutes but the need for manual skill has barely diminished over the years, and nowadays with the advent of minimal access techniques surgeons are being selected for something mysteriously called three-dimensional sense, which is not necessarily linked to verbal skill.

Other medical specialists – notably psychotherapists, as Jeremy Holmes shows in Chapter 18 – use words as their stock in trade. Although physicians and general practitioners do also rely on laboratory tests and drug treatments, many of them would agree that the ideal consultation is one in which the diagnosis is made entirely from the history and the patient is healed through dialogue alone. An 'invasive' intervention is seen as a last resort.

I do not wish to imply that surgeons do not listen or talk to their patients. I am merely pointing out that the surgeon's raison d'être is to operate, and that operating is done with the fingers, not the tongue. Surgeons are primarily craftsmen and from time immemorial craftsmen – whether sculptors, carpenters or potters – have let their fingers do the talking and have been economical with words.

Art versus craft versus science

Some surgeons feel that being called craftsmen is demeaning. It is more flattering to be called an artist or a scientist. Sir Michael Woodruff, in his inaugural lecture[3] in the Chair of Surgical Science at Edinburgh in 1957 said:

> Soon after arriving in Edinburgh I heard the view expressed that the university had committed an unpardonable gaffe in creating a Chair in a subject which does not exist. Surgery, I was told, is a craft, and surgical science is therefore a contradiction in terms.

111

Sir Michael argued persuasively that surgical science does exist (at least in the minds of professors of surgery), but as far as I know there are no chairs of surgical philosophy or surgical literature.

Scientists, with a few notable exceptions, tend to be numerate rather than literate. Medical science has currently been hijacked by mathematicians, and many of today's doctors feel that a concept has no validity unless it comes festooned with "p" values. Narrative, however, is an art. The craft of surgery lies somewhere between science, on one side, and art on the other. If surgeons aspire to be scientists rather than craftsmen they will tend to move away from art and narrative.

Gender issues

In Britain over 90% of consultant surgeons are men. The fact that there are only a few women in the specialty is often attributed to its career structure and to the attitudes of male consultant surgeons. These problems, however, afflicted all medical specialties only a few decades ago, and I think the real reason for the gender imbalance in surgery lies at a deeper level. Perhaps women are repelled by the cruelty referred to at the start of this chapter, and perhaps men are attracted by a specialty that began, centuries ago, as a part of military activity.

Narrative, by contrast, has a feminine bias. "Reading books" is listed as part of their leisure activity by 75% of teenage girls compared with 55% of boys.[4] Interestingly, in the past, literature, like surgery, was a male dominated field (the Bronte sisters used male pseudonyms when they began writing) but nowadays, of course, authors are at least as likely to be female as male.

Women have steadily broken into male bastions, including medicine, and the fact that surgery is one of the last redoubts may be due to factors more complex than male intransigence.

The surgeon as nerd

Surgery is a technical business and surgeons are interested in its minutiae. Chapter One in my copy of *Bailey and Love's Textbook of Surgery*[5] is entitled "Wounds and healing". Chapter 60 on page 1363 is entitled "The surgical patient" and is only three pages long. This is no bad thing. When I put myself in a surgeon's hands I want someone who has a deep and abiding interest in techniques of tying secure knots and who is happy to bore others to death with stories about great knots he has tied. In the same way, when my car breaks down I want a nerd who loves nuts and bolts rather than a philosopher who wonders whether I need a car at all or whether a spark plug knows it is a spark plug.

Emotional honesty

Narrative requires honesty about emotions, but the fact that operating involves inflicting mutilating and potentially painful wounds militates against the operator showing sensitivity. In theatre the surgeon has to be able to ignore everything except the job in hand. Before and after operating he cannot afford too much empathy. AJ Cronin in "Dr Finlay's Casebook" had his hero, immediately after Finals, apply for a post as assistant to a great surgeon. When asked why, Dr Finlay said: "You saved that poor woman's life. I want to do that." The great surgeon turned him down, telling him that with so much sympathy he was better suited to general practice.

In spite of these barriers, surgery and narrative share some common ground. Surgery, despite its military origins, is now fully a part of medicine. Surgeons and physicians share the same undergraduate education and in some cases become fellows of the same Royal College. As surgery requires less and less access, and endoscopists and radiologists become more and more interventionist, the traditional distinction between physician and surgeon is becoming blurred.[6]

Narrative based surgery?

The use of narrative in surgery is relevant to both training and clinical practice. Surgical narrative has some characteristic features, the most striking of which is brevity.

Training

Bailey and Love's Textbook of Surgery[5] is famous for its footnotes – succinct biographies of great surgeons of the past. These memorable one-liners are the apotheosis of surgical narrative. They could be dismissed as "mere anecdotes", but, as Jane Macnaughton points out in Chapter 20, anecdote has – or should have – a respectable place in clinical training, and surgery is no exception.

A surgeon gains experience one step at a time, and a story about someone else's case can be almost as helpful as going through the experience yourself (and less unpleasant, if the outcome was unfavourable).

Surgical audiences always enjoy hearing about challenging cases. In a meeting which includes scholarly lectures and scientific papers it is the case presentation that has the listeners on the edge of their seats. If the presenter stops at a crucial moment and asks: "What would you do now?" the question has a special urgency because a surgeon usually has to get the answer right first time.

Nevertheless the narrative of clinical case histories (as discussed in several other chapters of this book) is an indirect one compared to the immediate narrative of the consultation. The doctor telling the story cannot help "putting a spin on it", either to disguise the diagnosis or to justify his interpretation of the symptoms. All anecdote involves selection, which is perhaps why it has a bad name in medicine. Arguably, bias in the recall of surgical cases may be less of a problem than in those specialties where the management of the patient depends more heavily on nuance and outcomes are generally "softer".

Anecdotes are widely used to illuminate otherwise dull reports such as those of the defence societies or the Confidential Enquiries into Maternal Deaths.[7] We know instinctively that a clinical recommendation becomes more effective when it is illustrated by an example. I am not aware that formal research has been done on this but I suspect the effect is measurable. In this litigious age, however, published anecdotes lose much of their impact because details have to be omitted in attempts (usually futile) to preserve anonymity. If the importance of anecdote in education were better recognised and evaluated, we might be allowed to retain enough memorable detail to achieve maximum effect.

Listening

The first outpatient clinic I remember attending as a student was that of a kindly old surgeon. He told me to go and chat to a patient and he would follow in a few minutes. I protested that I had not yet been taught how to take a surgical history. "Just listen to him", he said. "Every patient has an interesting story to tell if only you can find out what it is".

Today I find myself saying the same thing to students, who look as disbelieving as I must have done. The longer a doctor practises, the more she/he lets the patient tell his or her story. What the surgeon does more than other doctors, I suspect, is to interrupt. Listening to the surgical patient is important. The main decision for a surgeon is whether or not to operate and unless the operation is life-saving this decision depends partly on the patient's character. Some patients have an unrealistic belief that an operation will change their lives and should be persuaded to try something else. For others, a surgical problem may mask a psychological one. One contemporary textbook suggests, for example, that more than half of women with menorrhagia may have depression,[8] and up to two-thirds of those with unexplained pelvic pain may be suffering the after-effects of physical or sexual abuse in childhood.[9]

Talking

Surgeons talk to patients as well as operating on them but explaining the details of the technical procedure hardly counts as narrative. What is important is not so much what the surgeon says as the way he says it. When television was introduced into the House of Commons, MPs were told that the most important aspects of their speech were how they looked, how they sounded and what they said, in that order.

Narrative is also, perhaps, too grand a word for the stories that a surgeon produces for colleagues. It is normally the task of the anaesthetist to maintain the oral narrative tradition in theatre. Victor Bonney, "the father of British gynaecology", gave some thought to how garrulous a surgeon should be while operating, in the preface to his classic textbook[10] first published in 1911:

> A surgeon should not gossip, for it is impossible for him to do his best work if he is continually engaged in irrelevant chatter; but a silent surgeon is unprofitable to those around him, for he should clearly outline the steps of the operation as it proceeds, and by apposite and instructive remarks compel the attention of those who are there to learn. It is the mark of a good operator to become more and more silent as the difficulty of the operation increases, of a bad one to become more loquacious.

Surgery based narrative

Though few surgeons are storytellers, many write well. Often they are sticklers for technical precision, paying proper attention to grammar, punctuation and the meaning of words. Surgeons tend to show more enthusiasm for factual subjects such as history than for poetry or magic realism.

As a subject for narrative by professional writers, surgery has pros and cons. On the plus side, it is physical and it makes people faint. Gritty truth has always been fashionable in narrative from Charles Dickens to Irving Welsh, and surgeons are in regular contact with blood and guts. The operating theatre is a place of drama, just as the courtroom is a useful setting for the lazy playwright.

Legal arguments, however, can be written in a way that the lay person can follow, whereas most operations are difficult to understand even with a full explanation. Indeed, surgery's main contribution to the narrative tradition may be its powerful imagery of masked people with your life in their hands. The surgeon's lightweight paper hat and mask are symbols as powerful as the judge's wig. Most surgeons know this and use them with discretion when not actually operating. It is just acceptable to wear them in the hospital corridor but even the most immature surgeon takes them off before driving home.

Surgery based narrative has had a powerful effect on the way British people view hospital doctors. One of the most potent of medical images was created by Richard Gordon and James Robertson Justice in the form of Sir Lancelot Spratt, senior surgeon at St Swithin's Hospital.[11] Watching the filmed version nowadays is an exercise in social history, with its obsequious patients and patrician consultants.

The film still influences attitudes, even today, and this creates problems for medical educators. Much of the good work of a medical school can quickly be undone when the students meet inappropriate role models on the wards. Some surgical trainees aspire to behave like Sir Lancelot but even for those who do not, there is subtle pressure to conform to the stereotype. Everyone now expects senior hospital doctors to be gruff, rich and rude to students, and for the newly appointed consultant the easiest response may be to go with the flow. Perhaps, after all, this is what patients secretly want.

———————◄❮❰❱❯►———————

1 Brock L. Surgery and Lister. *Ann Roy Coll Surg Eng* 1967; **40**: 55–64.
2 Diamond JC. *C: because cowards get cancer too ...* . London: Vermillion, 1998.
3 Woodruff M. *On science and surgery.* Edinburgh: University Press, 1977.
4 Central Statistical Office. *Social Trends, 1996* London: HMSO, 1996.

5 Rains AJH, Mann CV eds. *Bailey and Love's Short Practice of Surgery*, 20th edition. London: Lewis, 1988.

6 Porter R. Surgery. In: *The greatest benefit to mankind: a medical history of humanity from antiquity to the present*. London: Harper Collins, 1997, pp. 597–627.

7 Department of Health. Report on Confidential Enquiries into Maternal Deaths in the United Kingdom 1991–93. London: HMSO, 1996.

8 Iles S, Gath D. Psychological problems and uterine bleeding. *Bailliere's Clin Obstet Gynaecol* 1989; **3**: 75–89.

9 Drife J. The pelvic pain syndrome. *Brit J Obstet Gynaecol* 1993; **100**: 508–10.

10 Bonney V. General operative considerations. In: Howkins J, Stallworthy J eds *Bonney's Gynaecological Surgery*, 8th edition. London: Bailliere Tindall, 1974.

11 Gordon R. *Doctor in the House*. Harmondsworth: Penguin, 1961.

Dear Tom

Trisha Greenhalgh

Next week, you will be six years old. When I was your age, I already knew I wanted to become a doctor.

I went to medical school at Cambridge, where I learnt a lot of clever things about the human body. In Michaelmas term, 1978, we covered the anatomy, physiology and pathology of the brain. We dissected out parts with strange names like hippocampus and globus pallidus. We memorised the routes of all the tiny blood vessels that run in a chain around something called the Circle of Willis. We read about watershed zones and Berry aneurysms, and looked down microscopes at haemorrhagic and ischaemic infarcts.

A couple of years later, on a community medicine attachment, we studied the epidemiology of stroke. We talked about hypertension, smoking, diabetes, and thromboembolic disease, and we noted with some relief that the odds are stacked heavily against the elderly and those who are already ill. On our geriatric medicine firm, we admitted old people with strokes (declaring them "boring"), and once or twice, reluctantly, accompanied them on trips to the physiotherapy department.

In 1986, I took an important examination and was pleased that my long case was a stroke patient. My ability to locate the pathological lesion precisely in the left posterior inferior cerebellar artery from a meticulous assessment of which parts of the body the patient could still feel and move earned me the Membership of the Royal College of Physicians. The examiners congratulated me for knowing so much about strokes.

Tom, I am ashamed to say I believed them. Yet it was not until today that I learnt the most elementary lesson about cerebrovascular disease. When the choir had finished singing 'Abide With Me' and the congregation was sitting in deep reflective silence, your daddy picked you up and carried you to the coffin, and your faltering words, "Bye-bye mummy" echoed round the

118

little chapel, I finally understood some basic truths about this devastating condition.

If you ever go to medical school, Tom, tell the professors and lecturers to add a few facts to the core curriculum on the pathology of the human brain. Remind them to tell the students that cerebrovascular accidents are cruel and unfair, that they leave relationships broken and children motherless, and that the so-called risk factor profile often provides no satisfactory answers to the question, "why him?", "why her?" or "why me?"

Tell them that nature does not always protect the young, and that the task of rebuilding shattered lives is made no easier by a detailed knowledge of which vessel happened to burst on which side of the brain. Stroke prevention campaigns as currently formulated, even though based on the best available research evidence and using cost-effectiveness calculations that attach great value to the lives of people like your mummy, would not have saved her.

Meanwhile, Tom, I will copy this letter to the men and women of medical science. I will remind them that although they have made great strides in their research activities so far, there is no place for complacency when 5000 people of childbearing age still die or become seriously disabled from cerebrovascular disease in the UK every year.

Tom's mother died of a stroke in March 1998.

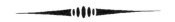

Learning and teaching narrative

13 Literature in medicine

Stephen Rachman

Where do we locate literature in medicine? What role does it play? What ends does it serve? These are questions that have been raised and addressed over the last three decades with increasing intensity by medical humanists, literary scholars, philosophers, ethicists, physicians, and writers. The answers are manifold. They range from the broad goal of using literature to facilitate the human-isation of medical perspective to the more specific exploration of the narrative aspects of medicine, which is the primary focus of this collection.

Literature has been used in medical instruction to promote moral and ethical reasoning, improve communication between doctor and patient, instill a deeper sense of medical history, explore the therapeutic value of storytelling, advance multicultural per-spectives, and increase self-consciousness on the part of medical practitioners.[1] And whether one is interested in using literature to promote any of these ends or merely to chasten an ambient or incipient sense of medical hubris, the need to locate literature in medicine is generally recognised as a corrective to this century's overvaluation of medical science and technology. Locating lit-erature in medicine proceeds from the recognition that "every aspect of medicine's history", as Charles Rosenberg has observed, "is necessarily 'social', whether acted out in laboratory, library, or at the bedside".[2] Medicine concerns itself with biological events, to be sure, but those events, once named, enter into language and, as such, are framed by culture and mediated by literature.

If scientific paradigms, as has been suggested by various critics, have sought to render language transparently neutral, and medi-cine has used the presumed transparency of scientific language to describe diseases and patients, then the study of literature makes the language of medicine, doctors, patients, and disease entities – the cultural frame of illness – visible once more.[3] In this sense, the function of literature in medicine is to restore language to our sight.

It may be recognised in the limitations of clinical description; the rhetoric of case studies; the polysemous quality of patient narratives; the growing social conscience of Tertius Lydgate in George Eliot's *Middlemarch*; the paternalistic rhetoric of Dr Kitteridge in Oliver Wendell Holmes's *Elsie Venner*; the disillusionment of Leo Tolstoy's Ivan Ilyich; the anti-authoritarian strategy of the mad narrator of Charlotte Perkins Gilman's *The Yellow Wallpaper*; or the astonishing play of pathological tropes in Ralph Waldo Emerson's *The Conduct of Life*.

The array of suitable literature – for example, doctors' stories, case studies, pathographies (illness narratives), novels, poems – is vast enough to make any choice appear arbitrary, and yet, taken singly or as a whole, works such as these call attention to the shared cultural terrain of literature and medicine – the relations among illness, health, language, and meaning.

The interdisciplinary merging of literature *and* medicine derives then from a cultural recognition that literature has always resided *in* medicine. In recent years, narrative has become the literary concept most powerfully and frequently invoked to explore this nexus. "Narrative", Suzanne Poirier has proposed, "is the 'glue' that holds literature and medicine together".[4] The work of Howard Brody, Rita Charon, Arthur W Frank, Kathryn Montgomery Hunter, and Arthur Kleinman have all helped to call attention to "the inherently narrative structure of medical knowledge and practice".[5] Virginia Woolf once noted that, given how common and profound illness is, it seemed "strange indeed that illness has not taken its place with love and battle and jealousy among the prime themes of literature".[6] At this juncture, it would be fair to say that literature, by way of the powerful explanatory models of narrative theory, has taken its place among the prime themes of medicine.

Narrative, of course, means story, and because stories may be fictional or true, written or oral, prose or verse, a wide array of narratives can be related to one another. Memoirs, medical case studies, and novels can all be compared with respect to their narrative properties. This has been particularly useful in examining sick roles, doctor–patient relationships, and applying, as Hunter suggests, "abstract knowledge to the care of the individual patient".[7] The study of narrative in medical contexts allows for focus on such elements as point of view; the relations among story, teller, and audience; levels of discourse. The telos of this type of analysis is to demonstrate the ways that knowledge is situated and relational, rooted in context, friable when extracted. In medicine, this means using narrative to mediate among doctor, patient, and illness.

For Howard Brody, narratives are squarely part of the therapeutic process. He argues that sickness disrupts personhood and suffering is produced and alleviated primarily by the meaning that one attaches to one's experience. It follows from this proposition that the organization of meaning involved in telling stories of sickness enables the reconstitution of the self.[8]

For Oliver Sacks, because many of his patients suffer from "anosagnosia" (difficulty in knowing or recognizing their own problems) involved in right-hemisphere disorders, observers have great difficulties imagining the inner state of the patient. Therefore, the clinical tale becomes a crucial device in filling the gap between patient and observer. In this sense, Sacks' task is to recover selves that appear to be lost to themselves. "We have each of us", Sacks writes, "a life-story, an inner narrative – whose continuity, whose sense, *is* our lives. It might be said that each of us constructs and lives, a 'narrative', and that this narrative is us, our identities".[9] Narrative has become the means *par excellence* for reconstituting the selfhood of the patient and therefore a key concept for finding literature in medicine.

But narrative is only one property of literature, not the whole of it, and in privileging it we should bear in mind the tensions in literary and medical perspectives. It remains an open question what productive relations exist between an understanding of symptoms, say, and a knowledge of tropes and rhetorical figures. This is not to say that metaphor or zeugma, for example, are irrelevant to the ways in which medical concepts are constructed. Oswei Temkin long ago pointed out the abiding power of metaphor in human biology, reminding us of the social connotations of such fundamental terms as "organism" from classical antiquity through the work of Rudolf Virchow.[10] It is perhaps most crucial to recognize both the literary and anti-literary aspects of medical thinking.

In *Illness as Metaphor*, perhaps the most widely-read essay on medicine and literature, Susan Sontag begins famously by declaring that "Everyone who is born holds dual citizenship, in the kingdom of the well and in the kingdom of the sick", and then proceeds to argue "that illness is *not* a metaphor, and that the most truthful way of regarding illness – and the healthiest way of being ill – is one purified of, most resistant to, metaphoric thinking".[11] Sontag effectively uses literature against itself. And while she plainly demonstrates how literary works have stigmatized cancer and tuberculosis through metaphoric treatment, abetting social or collective misunderstanding, it is equally plain that Sontag over-reaches: it is unavoidable that we assign meaning to disease.

Sontag blames the act of metaphorisation as well as the particular kinds of metaphors; and yet, we cannot escape metaphor and neither can she. Illness, by her lights, becomes a metaphoric kingdom replete with passports. The contradiction in her essay reflects the powerful tensions between literature and medicine, the play between restricted and open-ended meaning inherent in the predicament of illness and the process of healing.

The challenge of finding literature in medicine, of observing the literary texture of medicine, requires, therefore, a re-imagining of medicine, illness, and practice. It asks us to recognize the literary aspects of culture itself. "So for me", wrote William Carlos Williams,

> the practice of medicine has become the pursuit of a rare element which may appear at any time, at any place, at a glance. ... The relation between physician and patient, if it were literally followed, would give us a world of extraordinary fertility of the imagination which we can hardly afford. ... Do we not see that we are inarticulate? That is what defeats us. It is our inability to communicate to another how we are locked within ourselves, unable to say the simplest things of importance to one another. ... That gives the physician, and I don't mean the high-priced psychoanalyst, his opportunity. ... The physician enjoys a wonderful opportunity actually to witness the words being born. Their actual colors and shapes are laid before him carrying their tiny burdens. ... But after we have run the gamut of simple meanings that come to one over the years, a change gradually occurs ... a new meaning begins to intervene. For under that language to which we have been listening all our lives a new, a more profound language, underlying all the dialectics offers itself. It is what they call poetry.[12]

Words being born, language taking shape, these are the metaphysics of medical practice for Williams. Meaning is at once rooted in our corporeal existence and detached from it. As has been suggested, much has been made recently of the therapeutic value of writing and storytelling, the role of the voice in recovering the self disrupted by illness, but Williams' words remind us that the therapeutic scene, in its totality, yields a poetry, a language, a literature, finally.[13] Williams urges us to see and hear the literary quality that comprises the social and expressive core of medicine. It is not only that the practice of medicine is informed by literary understanding – by poetry – but that poetry is created in the practice of medicine.

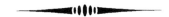

1 McLellan MF, Hudson Jones A. Why Literature and Medicine? *Lancet* 1996; **348**: 109–11. Montgomery Hunter K. Toward the Cultural Interpretation of Medicine, *Literature and Medicine* 1991; **10**: 1–17.

2 Rosenberg CE. Introduction Framing Disease: Illness, Society, and History. In: Rosenberg CE, Golden J eds *Framing Disease: Studies in Cultural History.* New Brunswick: Rutgers University Press, 1992; p. xiv.

3 Foucault M. *The Birth of the Clinic: An Archaeology of Medical Perception,* trans. A.M. Sheriden Smith. New York: Vintage Books, 1975. Most forcefully articulated the emergence of the transparent medical gaze in 18th-century French clinic, and the point has been reiterated in a variety of contexts by students of literature and medicine. See, for example, Charon R. To Build a Case: Medical Histories as Traditions in Conflict, *Literature and Medicine* 1992; **11**: 118–25. Weinstein A. The Unruly Text and the Rule of Literature. *Literature and Medicine* 1997; **16**: 2–3.

4 Poirier S. Toward a Reciprocity of Systems. *Literature and Medicine* 1991; **10**: 69.

5 Hudson Jones A. Literature and medicine: narrative ethics. *Lancet* 1997; **349**: 1243.

6 Woolf V. On Being Ill. *The Moment and Other Essays.* New York: Harcourt, Brace & World, 1948; p. 9.

7 Montgomery Hunter K. *Doctors' Stories: The Narrative Structure of Medical Knowledge.* Princeton: Princeton University Press, 1991; p. 47.

8 Brody H. *Stories of Sickness.* New Haven: Yale University Press, 1987; pp. 26–30.

9 Sacks O. *The Man Who Mistook His Wife For a Hat and Other Clinical Tales.* New York: Harper & Row: 1985; p. 110.

10 Temkin O. Metaphors of Human Biology. *The Double Face of Janus and Other Essays in the History of Medicine.* Baltimore: The Johns Hopkins University Press, 1977; pp. 271–83.

11 Sontag S. *Illness as Metaphor and AIDS and its Metaphors.* New York: Anchor Books, 1990; p. 3.

12 Carlos Williams W. The Practice. *The Doctor Stories.* New York: New Directions, 1984; pp. 123–5.

13 See for example, Frank AW, *The Wounded Storyteller: Body, Illness, and Ethics.* Chicago: University of Chicago Press, 1995, and Brody H. *Stories of Sickness.* New Haven: Yale University Press, 1987.

14 Teaching humanities in the undergraduate medical curriculum

Harriet A Squier

Why teach literature to undergraduate medical students?

The traditional medical school curriculum has focused on factual, rote learning about physiological processes and diseases. The kind of integrative, imaginative skills that a physician needs to actually apply the knowledge learned has only recently been recognised as something that can and should be taught to the doctor in training.[1-3] Large amounts of factual learning required by many medical schools, and the need to sacrifice their wider interests to make time for study, further constrict students' imaginative abilities.[4] Carefully selected, realistic readings chosen for their relevance to student experience and background can help bridge the gap between *knowing* the facts about the disease and *understanding* the patient's illness experience.[5 6] As the following two examples demonstrate, the study of literature can also help students to acknowledge and come to terms with the emotional aspects of their own professional involvement with patients and carers.

Case one

A class of second year medical students is required to undertake critical analysis of a selection of articles from medical journals. The tutor chooses three articles on the treatment and outcomes of hip fractures in the elderly. He wants the students to think about aspects of care that the authors of the research studies did not address, and how these omissions might have influenced patient outcomes and study results. The students in his small group discussion session stare at the articles and mumble that they look pretty complete to them. The tutor is frustrated that the students can't seem to do the assignment.

Commentary

These students have probably learned through hard experience that creative thinking is time consuming, produces few directly verifiable "facts" of the kind they have come to expect from other parts of the medical course, and is not rewarded with success in multiple choice exams. They have learned not to look beyond the page in front of them. In order to regain a sense of inquiry and restore students' confidence in using their imagination, the tutor asks them to read a short story related to the lives of elderly people.

In Ethan Canin's *We Are Nighttime Travelers,*[7] the reader becomes immersed in the lives of an elderly couple who have a number of health problems, and who are mired in the routine of 50 years of marriage. The husband, an outgoing and sociable retired salesman, starts reading and writing poetry and secretly delivers it to his wife in an attempt to rekindle their love. At the end of the story he coaxes his private and retiring wife outdoors for a midnight walk. They relive the feeling of courtship and romance they had long since forgotten, and feel reinforced in their ability to face the difficulties ahead.

Within the context of this story, students are asked to conjecture about the impact on this couple's life together if one of the pair should fall and break a hip. What would happen to the husband, considering his diabetes and other medical problems, if he should need surgery? What would be the effect on the physically stronger and healthier wife if she were the one who broke her hip? How might each react to the experience of nursing home care? What resources might be needed in order for either to return home?

The students are also asked to consider how their answers to such questions are supported by the text of the story. In this way, they are called upon to justify their *interpretive* responses to a piece of fiction in the same way as they have, in other classes, been required to justify factual responses to physiological or clinical assignments.

The students are then invited to return to their original set of medical journal articles and critique them in terms of how they

129

might influence the care of this specific elderly couple. The tutor broadens the discussion to include speculation about other common problems in the elderly, such as dementia, social isolation, lack of caregiver support, and so on. Finally, the group is invited to return to the original task set by the tutor, to see if, in the light of the discussion that has occurred, they can now think of aspects of the problem (hip fracture) which the research articles failed to address.

Case two

When asked to instruct a new mother about breastfeeding, a third year medical student responds by giving a detailed explanation of the biochemical composition of breast milk. The mother looks perplexed, and by the end of the interaction, still does not understand why the medical student is encouraging her to breastfeed when the bottle sounds so much easier.

Commentary

This student is unable to imagine what a new mother needs to know in order to make an informed decision about breastfeeding. Moreover, the complex cultural, psychological and socioeconomic issues that underpin personal health choices are hidden to this student and appear not to have been covered or understood in the medical course up to now.

With the specific goal of improving both empathy with patients and the quality of advice given to new mothers, students on this attachment are asked to read "Milk", a short story about a middle class white woman who is convalescing in hospital after a caesarean section.[8] The woman in the next bed, an African Caribbean from a socioeconomically deprived neighbourhood, is suspicious of official medical care and advice, and chooses not to breastfeed her child. The story describes how the premature black infant rapidly becomes ill and dies from gastroenteritis, and includes first-person narrative by the middle class mother who cannot understand her room-mate's decision to bottlefeed.

The story also contains some powerful dialogues between patients and professionals, exposing racial discrimination and dismissal of the black mother's own concerns about her child. The narrator (the white mother) expresses confusion and despair at the death of the black infant, a response that is perhaps symbolic of that of the health professional whose "evidence based" advice is repeatedly unheeded for unfathomed sociocultural reasons.

Inexperienced students often find it impossible to engage with the illness experiences and health choices of a patient in a hospital bed. But this fictional story about two mothers from different cultural backgrounds, one of whom sees her baby die, generally sparks lively small group discussion on a range of different features of the story. Issues such as patient empowerment, access to medical care for different social, ethnic, or other disadvantaged groups, and the importance of cross-cultural understanding, tend to be central themes in their discussions.

In this exercise, students are then invited to look specifically at the factors influencing a mother's decision to breastfeed, and to relate the broad discussion on socioeconomic, psychological and ethnographic themes which they have just had to preliminary readings they have done before the session (on breastfeeding statistics and the objective risks and benefits of different feeding methods). They are then encouraged to discuss how they might broach the topic with real patients from different ethnic back-grounds, who, like the patient in the story, may mistrust the medical system the students represent.

In both these examples, the readings offered to the students have a transferable lesson that goes beyond particular medical conditions – that patient-relevant outcomes of illness episodes or health promotion initiatives depend largely on socioeconomic realities and upon psychological or cultural features of each case. It might seem superficially desirable to match items of recommended literature with the particular medical topic the students are discussing, but it should be remembered that unlike diseases, literature cannot be easily distilled into lists of discrete issues or solutions. Indeed, the chief value of literature is the inherent complexity and holism of the story medium which reflects the complexity of real people living real lives, thereby allowing the student to reach a deeper and more comprehensive appreciation of the patient's predicament.

The literature and medicine course at Michigan State University, USA

Michigan State University has offered a one-month course in medical humanities since the early 1990s. Students select either history, literature, or spirituality and spend 2 hours a week on this option for 4 weeks. Students taking the literature option are offered weekly study units which cluster several short contemporary literary works around a central theme in order to explore multiple perspectives on these topics. Students may choose from Women and Medicine; Doctors and Patients; Illness and the Meaning of Disease; Ageing, Dying and Grief; and Medicine, Minorities, and Culture.

Creative writing exercises are undertaken in which a literary work is rewritten from a new perspective, at least one from the point of view of someone of a different race, gender, or age from the student. In their discussion and writing, students generally display high levels of empathy toward others, moral reasoning, and tolerance toward divergent interpretations and unsympathetic characters.

Another input of literature to the Michigan State medical curriculum has been in the doctor–patient relationship course (see Case two above). Students read and discuss clusters of short contemporary works around such issues as what patients look for in doctors, what it means to be ill, culture and healing, what it means to be a doctor, and effective and ineffective doctor–patient interactions. In the large group setting, students listen to patients, physicians, and healers telling their stories; they then practise "interviewing" family members and classmates and discuss the methods used to elicit their stories. Despite the inductive learning style, where students are not told what the "right" answers are, we have found that around 90% of students portray either patient-centered or relationship-centered models in this exercise by the end of a 7-week course.

Developing a literature and medicine curriculum

Approximately 30% of American medical schools include some kind of instruction in literature and medicine.[9] Many of these courses are elective (optional) modules, usually lasting one semester (part time for half a year), and offer a variety of readings (including novels, plays, poems, and short stories) around a wide range of different topics. Shorter courses are also offered at some colleges, and there is a variable degree of integration of literature and the humanities into the mainstream medical curriculum.

The basics of curriculum design need to be meticulously applied to literature and medicine curricula in order to develop a learner-centered, relevant programme, and to improve the chances that the course will be incorporated into the mainstream curriculum. These basics include determining needs, setting clear goals and objectives, assessing students formally against course objectives, designing appropriate and achievable assignments for written assessments, allocating adequate resources (including tutors and their training), and evaluating the content and overall outcomes of the course.[10]

Determining needs. A course that is well-intentioned, but that does not match the needs, backgrounds, or experiences of the learners, may be doomed to failure.[11] It is essential that characteristics of the learners, including their needs, learning style, past experiences, and existing knowledge and skills be considered in the course design. Skills and experience acquired on previous courses or in jobs held before or during medical school should be used as a resource and built upon, rather than simply reiterated. In general, however, it should not be assumed that the typical student on a foundation level literature and medicine module will have well developed skills in the identification of personal emotion, verbal communication, or explication of narrative.

Course goals, which refer to the academic faculty's desired (or required) outcomes and reasons for the course, should always be kept in mind when making choices about specific course objectives, content, and evaluation. If the goal of a course is to further student understanding of patient and physician perspectives as part of the doctor–patient relationship course, asking students to discuss the uses of metaphors in a story or rhythm and alliteration in a poem may not advance, and may even divert attention from, this broad goal. On the other hand, if the goal is to develop a deeper understanding of how humans communicate, this kind of literary discussion may well be appropriate. Other examples of goals are shown in Box 14.1.

Course objectives refer to the specific knowledge, skills, behaviours, or attitudes that students are to acquire by the end of the course. These objectives should be achievable, demonstrable, and student oriented, and tend to be described in terms of a measurable performance. For example, words such as "compare and contrast", "hypothesise", "analyse", "imagine", "conjecture",

---

Box 14.1: Examples of goals for a literature and medicine course for undergraduates

- To further student understanding of patient and physician perspectives as part of a doctor–patient relationship course.
- To prepare and motivate students for consultation skills training.
- To prepare students for their clinical years by improving their understanding of psychosocial issues and developing empathy for patients.
- To develop a deeper understanding of how humans communicate.
- To stimulate self-reflection and moral imagination.

"describe", "defend", or "facilitate" are appropriate things which students might be expected to *do* at the end of the course, and indicate the higher order learning that should occur in inductive, learner centered education.[12] Typical course objectives are shown in Box 14.2.

Clearly, objectives need to be tailored to students' baseline competence and the overall goals of the course. Students who are just beginning their clinical attachments will be unable to apply what they learn to actual patient care experiences since they have had so few of these; conversely, more senior students will become frustrated if they are not given time and opportunity to reflect on their clinical experiences with patients and integrate these with the material presented on the course.

Formal assessment of any taught course must be linked to course objectives. For example, if you have set as an objective that

---

Box 14.2: Examples of objectives for a literature and medicine course for undergraduates

By the end of this course, students should be able to

- discuss the differences between the biomedical model of disease and the biopsychosocial model of illness;
- portray through an appropriate creative medium their view of the ideal doctor–patient relationship;
- hypothesise how changing the point of view of a story would change the events depicted and/or the interpretation of these events;
- reflect on and compare a fictional story with a real experience they have had with a patient.

---

students should demonstrate empathy, you will need to somehow document whether or not they have done so. Although the demonstration of empathy may seem a "soft" outcome,[13] students' ability to express empathy with characters and with their classmates, as well as their ability to listen carefully to their classmates and facilitate discussion, can be readily documented when observing small group discussions.

Written assignments serve educational as well as evaluative roles in literature and medicine courses, and can allow for personal, creative expression. It is important to avoid an excessive focus on the grading of students' written assignments as this may create perverse incentives (for example, to reproduce a "right" answer) and defeat the overall goals of the course. Since a feeling of safety is necessary for students to risk self reflection, interpretation, and creativity, grading should encourage rather than discourage these behaviours. Fine distinctions between students is not a desirable goal of grading creative or imaginative writing in this context. Instead, evaluators should give positive feedback and use probing or thought-provoking comments to encourage reflection.

Resources for the course should include seminar rooms for small group discussion, study packs or books, and sufficient experienced tutors for small group facilitation. Course literature should include clearly focused discussion questions for students and their tutors to address, as well as guidance for tutors on the specific goals for each class. These should identify the point of the exercise and how it relates to the clinical problem or case vignette.

Tutor training and orientation. One of the biggest barriers to introducing a new module in the medical curriculum is resistance from medical tutors who may fail to appreciate the potential value of the proposed change. As with any other curriculum change, those who actually teach the students must agree that there is a curricular need for the new course, and feel that the proposed change will advance their personal teaching goals.

Training sessions, facilitated by the course director, in which course tutors discuss a particular reading amongst themselves should help them gain ownership of the material and improve the confidence of those with little previous experience in teaching literature. These steps also help to ensure similar learning experiences across multiple small groups and allow tutors to appreciate and modify the teaching design. As with all small group seminars, thorough preparation and competent facilitation will greatly increase the effectiveness of small group sessions.

135

Course outcomes may be difficult to evaluate using standard checklists designed for the more biomedical modules in the curriculum. It is better to consider asking students specific questions that assess how well they feel they mastered the course objectives, and how effective the readings, discussion, and writing assignments were in helping them achieve this. For material that is being offered for the first time, students and tutors should be asked to assess in detail the utility of each of the readings, the reading questions, and the written assignments as well as the overall unit design. The responses provide essential feedback for revisions. All of this information, plus analysis of student written assignments to demonstrate the acquisition of knowledge, skills and attitudes, can provide useful feedback for administrative bodies.

Ideally, we should document that literature and medicine courses result in changes in student behaviours. Currently the techniques necessary for this kind of documentation are not widely known or used, and the objective measurement of behavioural outcomes is still at the developmental stage. Possible measures could consist of a pre-assessment given before a course, to evaluate students' empathic abilities, narrative analysis, or understanding of patient issues. The same instrument would be given after the course to document improvement. Alternatively, student behaviour with standardised patients or on videotaped interviews could be compared to assess improvement. Ultimately, documentation that humanities training does, indeed, improve clinical performance will solidify the place of medical humanities in the medical school curriculum. The innovative medical humanities course in Sydney University is now an established part of the curriculum that is formally examined.[14]

Overcoming barriers

An individual who takes on the task of introducing humanities into the medical school curriculum faces many barriers, including philosophical, institutional, attitudinal, and personal. One reason medical humanities may be difficult to sell to medical school administrations and teaching faculty is that the method of learning in medical humanities is very different from typical medical education strategies. Students' usual activities are task oriented: if they need to know the nerves of the brachial plexus, they memorize them. If they need to manage diabetic ketoacidosis, they follow a formula for calculating the dosage of insulin, infusion rates, potassium supplementation, etc., write the orders, then wait to see what happens. In both these examples, success (or failure) is directly and objectively measurable.

This task orientation has characterized medical practice for decades. In the 19th century, counting pulses, titrating dosages of medicines, charting fevers, and observing microbes through newly invented microscopes enhanced the physician's sense of expertise and professionalism at a time when medicine and quackery could be hard to distinguish. The reliance on scientific observation, classification, and measurement and the sense of mastery associated with these activities, continues to define the parameters of much of medical practice.

Humanities education directly challenges the scientific certainty that underpins Western medicine, by valuing subjective knowledge alongside the objective, inductive reasoning alongside deductive, and human experience and emotion alongside scientific data. Indeed, other authors in this book have explored the somewhat heretical notion that medical thinking and the process of practice very often fit a narrative, rather than a hypothetico-deductive, paradigm. There is, in addition, a growing body of evidence that treatment outcomes may improve simply by improving the interaction between doctors and patients.[15] Such studies challenge the notion that it is the content of the physician's intervention that cures the patient, and promote the importance of "healing behaviour" as a style of practice – an approach which lends itself to a humanities framework for teaching and learning.

In the absence of "hard outcomes" on medical humanities courses, perhaps the best marketing tool for "selling" the idea of such a course is the subjective success and popularity of existing courses in other institutions. In its first offering, the medical humanities curriculum at Michigan State received the highest student evaluations of any course in the second year curriculum. In some places, medical humanities has been offered initially as an elective, or even non-credit, option and proved so popular (with consistently positive evaluations by students and tutors) that the medical administration has been persuaded to convert the elective course into a for-credit or even compulsory course.[16]

There is, in addition, a growing societal desire for more humanistic and socially responsive patient care which has prompted bodies such as the Association of American Medical Colleges (AAMC) to call for medical school training that is relevant, rather than merely extensive.[17] Rather than seeing humanities training in opposition to science training, the AAMC Medical Schools Objectives Project has declared humanities training as necessary for teaching the application of science to individual patients as well as to needy populations.

Conclusion

The study of literature encourages higher order learning and the development of empathy, imagination, self knowledge, and moral reflection. Carefully crafted courses, which provide relevant readings in a safe environment, improve student motivation, attention to and understanding of language, and promote the ability to integrate scientific knowledge with patient interaction. While barriers to medical humanities education do exist, there is currently unprecedented opportunity to introduce new courses and to integrate literature into the mainstream medical curriculum.

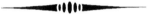

1 Smith BH, Taylor RJ. Medicine – a healing or a dying art? *Brit J Gen Pract* 1996; **46**: 249–51.

2 Weatherall D. *Science and the Quiet Art: Medical Research and Patient Care.* Oxford: Oxford University Press, 1995.

3 General Medical Council. *Tomorrow's Doctors. Recommendations for Undergraduate Medical Education.* London: General Medical Council, 1993.

4 Jackson M. Medical humanities in medical education. *Medical Education* 1996; **30**: 395–6.

5 McManus IC. Humanity and the medical humanities. *Lancet* 1995; **346**: 1143–5.

6 Downie RS. Literature and Medicine. *J Med Ethics* 1991; **17**: 93–8.

7 Canin E. We are nighttime travelers. From *Emperor of the air.* New York: Harper & Row, 1989.

8 Pollack E. Milk. In: Henderson W. (ed.). *Best of the small presses.* Wainscott, NY: Pushcart, 1995.

9 Hunter KM, Charon R, Coulehan JL. The study of literature in medical education. *Acad Med* 1995; **70**: 787–94.

10 Kemp JE. *Instructional Design: A plan for unit and course development.* Belmont, CA: Fearon-Pitman Publishers, 1977.

11 Borgenicht L. For this they go to medical school: student reactions to "Heartsounds". *The Pharos of Alpha Omega Alpha,* Summer 1983; **46**(3): 32–6.

12 Almy TP, Colby KK, Zubkoff M, Gephart DS, Moore West M, Lundquist LL. Health, society and the physician. Problem based learning of the social sciences and humanities. Eight years of experience. *Ann Int Med* 1992; **116**: 569–74.

13 Moore FD. Criteria of humanity. Defining the indefinable. *Ann Surg* 1985; **201**: 231–2.

14 Cossart Y, Pegler M (eds). *Doctor! Look behind you.* Sydney: University of Sydney, 1993. pp. 3–31.

15 Stewart M, Brown JB, Weston WW, McWhinney IR, McWilliam CL, Freeman TR. *Patient-centered medicine: transforming the clinical method.* Thousand Oaks, CA: Sage Publications, 1995.

16 Abbey L. Personal correspondence, 10/1/97.
17 AAMC. Oral presentation, Medical Schools Objective Project. AAMC Annual Meeting, Washington, DC, 1997.

15 The golden narrative in British medicine

Stuart Hogarth and Lara Marks

> Before commencing the study of the symptoms, [the doctor] will inform himself of the age and profession of the subject; of his habitual state of embonpoint or of emaciation, of strength or of weakness, of health or of disease; of the affections under which he has labored previously to the present, of his good or bad conformation.
>
> *Pierre Louis. Essay on Clinical Instruction, 1832*[1]

> It is often very satisfying to the sick to be allowed to tell, in their own way, whatever they deem important for you to know. Give a fair, courteous hearing, and, even though Mrs Chatterbox, Mr Borum, and Mrs Lengthy's statements are tedious, do not abruptly cut them short, but endure and listen with respectful attention, even though you are ready to drop exhausted.
>
> *Daniel Cathell. The Physician Himself from Graduation to Old Age, 1924*[2]

Something of the history of the troubled relationship between patient and healer is neatly encapsulated in the different attitudes of Louis and Cathell. For Louis, the patient's account of his medical history is central to the diagnostic process. For Cathell, by contrast, it is the social and therapeutic roles of narratives which are important; listening to the patient is a form of professional courtesy and gives pleasure to the sick but it is not, he implies, of great diagnostic value. The question historians must ask is to what extent these contrasting attitudes, separated by nearly a century of dramatic developments in medical knowledge and practice, illustrate perennial ambiguities and tensions in the doctor–patient relationship, and to what extent they suggest a fundamental transformation in that relationship and a corresponding shift in the clinical status and role of the patient's narrative.[3][4]

The history of diagnostic techniques during this period would certainly suggest a dramatic change in the clinical status of sickness narratives. Indeed the history of diagnosis in the last two centuries has been broadly understood by many historians as a proliferation of techniques for eliciting clinical data directly from the bodies of the sick, with a corresponding diminution in the importance of patients' attempts to render into language their experiences of pain and discomfort.* As medicine learnt to listen and look at the body in new and powerful ways its focus of attention shifted; it ceased in consequence to grant stories of the sick such close attention. But this has not always been the case.[5-7]

Until the 18th century, physicians based a large part of their diagnosis on what their patients told them.[8] Physical examination was limited to pulse taking, further investigation of the body relying more on the analysis of excreta (the mantula or urine flask having been the trademark of the medical profession since the medieval period). The importance of the patient's words is most powerfully exemplified by the practice of epistolary medicine, in which diagnosis and treatment were carried out entirely by letter.[9] Historians have sought to locate this humanist and person-centred medicine in its social and economic context: in this period a variety of medical practitioners competed for the business of the sick. Establishing a medical practice was dependent on winning the confidence of patients: paying customers expecting value for money, or powerful patrons who naturally treated their physicians as clients. Professional success therefore required social skills, gravitas, good manners and, above all, the ability to listen. Gaining the trust of the patient made business as well as clinical sense.[10 11]

By the late 18th century a new kind of doctor–patient relationship was emerging in another context – the hospital. Here the balance of power between doctor and patient started to alter.[12] Doctors, dealing with large numbers of poor patients, began classifying and labelling disease in a new way. With the development of pathological anatomy and new techniques of physical examination, doctors were able to probe into the patient's body directly and thereby became less reliant upon the patient's narrative. The development of thermometers (1700s), stethoscopes (1819), ophthalmoscopes (1850), and laryngoscopes (1855), accelerated this process. By the 1870s many physicians believed that inventions such as these meant that "the physiological forces expressing health and disease could be measured precisely"[13] and

---

* This chapter will deal with a period of dramatic change – the 18th through to the 20th centuries. Prior to this period, diagnostic practice (based on the Classical Galenic system of medicine) changed relatively little.

could anounce that "thermometer readings were beyond the control of the patient's will, or of extraneous circumstances, and thus were unerringly accurate". A commitment to scientific objectivity, based upon the increasing authority of quantitative over qualitative evidence, was beginning to emerge in medicine.[14]

Traditionally, historians have linked the decline of the patient's narrative with the rise of hospital medicine. It is not that doctors stopped listening to patients' stories at this time, but in hearing what patients had to say they were no longer trying to understand the unique histories of individuals. They searched instead for what may have been the common characteristics of the same disease in different people. The role of the case history became counter-balanced by a new form of clinical knowledge developed in the hospital.

Prior to the 19th century, medical knowledge envisaged sickness holistically, as a deviation from an individual's unique natural state. The new hospital paradigm classified illness according to morbid ideal types derived from observation and comparison of large numbers of cases. The "sick man" was thus reconceptualised as "the accident of his disease, the transitory object upon which it happens to have seized".[15]

At the same time as generating a new kind of knowledge and practice, the hospital helped to create a new form of doctor – one who began to combine the previously separate skills of the surgeon and the apothecary. Known as the general practitioner, this new kind of doctor highlighted tensions within medical practice in this period. In institutional settings the general practitioner might practise the more depersonalised type of medicine, but as a family doctor, his practice had to be based upon an intimate knowledge of patients' lives and circumstances.[16-19] As other chapters in this book suggest, the varying emphasis today placed upon patient narrative by different strata of the medical profession became apparent in the 19th century.

The new role of family doctor, trusted friend and confidant, was in large part a service provided for the rapidly expanding middle-classes. As long as medical treatment has been a commodity to be bought and sold, the quality of treatment has varied according to the social status of patients. The rich, whose money can command the attentive ear of an elite physician have always been listened to respectfully. Poor patients, on the other hand, have often been less well served.[20] Take, for example, the story told by Kate Taylor, born in Packenham, Suffolk in 1891, the fourteenth of fifteen children, who recalled the death of one of her sisters at the turn of the 19th century.

> Margery left school before she was thirteen, and went as general servant at the local grocery shop. The snobbery of those days was unbelievable. The woman couldn't afford a servant and paid only 1 shilling a week, and Mother had to do Margery's washing. Poor Margery was overworked and underfed, and her living and sleeping quarters were dark and damp. Margery was allowed home for two hours once a week. One evening she came home and letting her hands fall into her lap, she said to Mother "I feel just like that." Mother could see she was ill. I was sent to the shop to say that Margery wasn't well and could not return that evening, to which the wretched woman replied, "Tell her to be early in the morning." However, she was too ill to get up in the morning and I was sent to Ixworth to the doctor. He gave me a bottle of Epsom salts. He didn't come to see her, and in ten days she was dead. Father went for the certificate from the doctor and to the relieving officer for an order for a parish coffin. The doctor signed the certificate stating diphtheria as the cause of death. He hadn't seen her. Of course, it was pneumonia. Because of the doctor's statement of diphtheria, the coffin was not allowed in the church. There were just committal prayers at the graveside. After these were said Mother looked straight at the vicar and said to him, "You have kept her out of church, you can't keep her out of heaven."[21]

This story of neglect of Kate's sister is a poignant 20th century example of the level of care which the poor could expect from their doctors. As far back as the 18th century, medical theorists and moral philosophers had argued that sensibility was class-specific; that sensitivity to one's surroundings and body was a product of one's social status. There was scepticism on the part of doctors about the poor's ability to give an accurate or useful account of their illness. One doctor, John Rutherford, who was based at the Edinburgh Royal Infirmary, complained that many of his hospital patients were "poor people and many of them so indolently ignorant that they can give no account of the rise and progress of their diseases".[22] In the 19th century this distrust of the poor patient was extended to all women patients, who were characterised as hysterical by many medical men.[23]

It is unsurprising that the sick have often voted with their feet, opting for medical practitioners who offer them time and space to talk. As early as the 1840s alternative practitioners, such as herbalists, homeopaths, and mesmerists were able to expand their businesses rapidly on the basis of reputations gained for listening to clients.[24] Today's alternative practitioners continue this tradition and offer in addition a variety of medical cosmologies which all tend to place the "patient self" at the centre of the consultation and therapy.

It could be argued that, in the 20th century the growth of medical technology, state health provision, and more recently, the rise of evidence based medicine, have all tended to reinforce the diminishing importance of the patient narrative in the understanding of health and sickness.[25] However, the importance of narrative has not been totally eclipsed. Within the medical profession a number of practitioners have called for patient-centred approaches to the clinical process. In part this has been an expression of the belief of many doctors that they practise a clinical art in which sensitivity to the patient as a person is fundamental.[26] Around the beginning of this century, a renewed emphasis on the need to listen to the patient arose, gaining impetus from the emerging disciplines of psychoanalysis and psychology. At the same time as new diagnostic technologies such as X-rays were increasing doctors' reliance on instrumental aids to diagnosis, medical practitioners were also being urged to improve their skills as empathic listeners.[27] The beginning of the second half of the 20th century saw a similar process take hold in general practice; at a time when general practitioners first gained increased access to powerful diagnostic and investigative facilities providing effective scientific back-up to their work, Michael Balint was helping them to appreciate that two narratives intersect in complicated ways within medical consultations, the patient's and the doctor's. This perception encouraged a humanistic and reflective approach to the clinical encounter and became particularly influential in the postgraduate training of general practitioners (see Chapters 1 and 11).

Doctors' narratives

So far we have looked at patients' narratives, but what of those created by medical practitioners? At a time when doctors were growing sceptical about the stories of their patients, they were also devising new techniques for recording their own stories. In the 19th century, the case history, hitherto usually kept for the doctor's own reference or for educational purposes, became increasingly central to clinical practice. Coincident with the rise in new diagnostic tools was the standardisation of medical record keeping, particularly in hospitals and other institutional settings. Looked at broadly, far from eliminating the narrative, new techniques of examination (linked as they were to new bureaucratic standards of documentation) transformed the patient narrative into a case history that became the cornerstone of institutionalised welfare.

Prisoners, students, lunatics and paupers all found the details of their lives being meticulously recorded by officials.[28] New forms of social relations were arising in medicine, based less on personal knowledge of individuals and more on generalisations about categories of persons. The process of standardisation which ensued created its own problems: while officials complained that the information given to them by inmates could be confusing, the records kept by doctors could be equally baffling not only to their patients but also to their medical colleagues. Consider for example, the experiences of Bella Aaronovitch who suffered terrible complications as a result of an operation for appendicitis in 1928. From 1928 to 1932 Bella underwent numerous treatments and operations and when finally recovering was released only to suffer walking problems for 13 years. After a couple of years of bearing her walking difficulties she attempted to get help:

> The following week I went back to see the doctor. He read the report about me and not surprisingly looked a trifle vague. My hospital notes were very long and probably detailed, though they were never co-ordinated, with the result that if information was required by another doctor, it gave a not too accurate account of the different hospitals I had been in, complete with the number of operations and ended with the words, "Now apparently quite better and able to work".
>
> To have to unravel a five-year history of illness where cause and effect were so inextricably interwoven, made it difficult to reduce this maze of information to manageable proportions. It was also a question of being interested enough. I know from experience that most doctors hate to be confronted with cases of this kind. They have no direct knowledge of the original illness and have to obtain the information from reports and what the patients happen to know about themselves; all this is very time-consuming and open to misinterpretation.[29]

Bella's story, like that of Kate Taylor, suggests that whatever doctors have made of the stories they are told, the sick themselves have continued to create their own personal meanings from experiences of illness and health. Indeed, not all the stories that patients tell about their experiences of health are primarily medical in meaning or purpose. Narratives of suffering and redemption, for instance, have been an important literary form in religious settings. The sick have continued to place their pain, suffering, disability, and fear of death within the context of their wider lives, their family history and working conditions, their access to the necessities of life. Insufficient recognition of this rich narrative context lies behind the frustration expressed by the Enlightenment historian, George Rousseau, when he writes: "if more historians of medicine studied autobiography, they might better understand the case history".[30]

Awareness that narratives of sickness exist outside, and are indeed generally being formed prior to the consulting room, is important for understanding the wider context of the clinical encounter. In the 19th century the religious autobiography with its narratives of sin and salvation remained important whilst secular autobiographies proliferated and moved down the social scale to encompass the whole of society – no longer the preserve of statesmen and soldiers, secular autobiography was taken up by the working classes to tell their own stories.[31][32]

The 19th century can also be seen as a period in which the patient took on a heightened social significance: viewed through the lens of Romanticism, tuberculosis, for instance, became a signifier of artistic temperament. As the sick role became more established in Victorian culture so sickness narratives took on greater significance.[33] In their autobiographies great men and women like Charles Darwin and Harriet Martineau recounted their physical suffering alongside their professional successes.[34][35] Imaginative literature, too, succumbed to the new trend: "There is scarcely a Victorian fictional narrative without its ailing protagonist, its depiction of a sojourn in the sickroom".[36] Narratives of sickness thus came to play an important role in Victorian culture generally. In the case of autobiographies by invalids, the chronically and the acutely sick, this has evolved in the 20th century into a discrete genre.[37]

Conclusion

Whether taking place in the 17th or 20th century, the dialogue between the doctor and the patient has always been at the heart of the clinical encounter. Nonetheless, in the construction of health and illness there remains a tension between what the doctor and the patient see as important. The complexity of the contemporary patient–doctor relationship reflects the multiple changes that have occurred in medical knowledge and practice over time. Embedded in these developments are changes in the relative social and economic status of medical practitioners and the sick.

The declining importance of the narrative to modern medicine can be traced to hospitals for the poor in the late 18th century. A new understanding of disease as physicochemical disruption allowed disease to be identified and dealt with in ways that heeded little attention to the stories of the sick. By contrast, a renewed emphasis on narrative in the late 20th century can be linked to the declining power of professionals and the reconceptualisation of patients as complex individuals powerfully conditioned by familial and early childhood experiences on the one hand, and as consumers with demands and rights on the other. Though the patient's narrative may have declined, it has by no means fallen.

Narrative based medicine has a history and, as the other chapters in this book suggest, it also has a future.

Acknowledgment

We would like to thank Dr Brian Hurwitz for his contributions to our thinking on how to approach this chapter, and for pointing us towards some helpful historical sources.

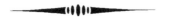

1 Louis P. *Essay on clinical instruction.* London: S. Higley, 1832.
2 Cited in: Shorter E. *Primary care.* In: Porter R ed. *The Cambridge Illustrated History of Medicine.* Cambridge: Cambridge University Press, 1996, p. 145.
3 Porter D and Porter R. *Patients' progress: doctors and doctoring in eighteenth-century England.* Cambridge: Polity Press, 1989.
4 Wear A. *History of the doctor–patient relationship.* Euro America, Ishikayu, 1995.
5 Reiser SJ. *Medicine and the reign of technology.* Cambridge: Cambridge University Press, 1978.
6 Reiser SJ. The decline of the clinical dialogue. *J Med Philos.* 1978; **3**: 305–13.
7 Reiser SJ. The science of diagnostic technologies. In: Bynum WF, Porter R eds *The companion encyclopaedia to the history of medicine,* Volume 2. London: Routledge, 1993, pp. 826–51.
8 Nicholson M. The art of diagnosis. In: Bynum WF, Porter R eds *The companion encyclopaedia to the history of medicine,* Volume 2. London: Routledge, 1993, pp. 801–25.
9 Nicholson M. The art of diagnosis: medicine and the five senses. In: Porter D, Porter R eds. *Patient's progress: doctors and doctoring in eighteenth-century England.* Cambridge: Polity Press, 1989, pp. 72–8.
10 Jewson ND. Medical knowledge and the patronage system in eighteenth-century England. *Sociology* 1974; **8**: 369–85.
11 Jewson ND. The disappearance of the sick man from medical cosmology. *Sociology* 1976; **10**: 225–44.

12 Waddington I. The role of the hospital in the development of modern medicine: a sociological analysis. *Sociology* 1973; **7**: 211–24. For a local study see also Fissell M. *Patients, power and the poor in eighteenth century Bristol.* Cambridge: Cambridge University Press, 1991, especially Chapter 8.

13 Reiser SJ. *Medicine and the reign of technology.* Cambridge: Cambridge University Press, 1978, pp. 118–19.

14 Trohler U. To improve the evidence of medicine: arithmetic observation in clinical medicine in the eighteenth and early nineteenth centuries. In: *History and Philosophy of the Life Sciences,* 1998; **10**(Suppl.): 31–40.

15 Foucault M. *Birth of the clinic.* London: Allen Lane, 1973, p. 59.

16 Loudon I. The Concept of the Family Doctor. *Bull History Med.* 1984; **LVIII**: 347–62.

17 Loudon I. *Medical care and the general practitioner.* Oxford: Clarendon Press, 1986, pp. 275–9.

18 Shorter E. *Doctors and their patients, a social history.* New Brunswick: Transaction, 1991.

19 Digby A. *Making a medical living: doctors and their patients in the English market for medicine, 1720–1911.* Cambridge: Cambridge University Press, 1994.

20 Fissell M. The Decline of the Patient's Narrative. In: French R, Wear A eds *British Medicine in an Age of Reform.* London: Routledge, 1991, pp. 92–109.

21 Taylor K. Destiny. In: Burnett J ed. *Obscure autobiographies of childhood, education and family from the 1820s–1920s.* London: Penguin, 1982, p. 293.

22 Rutherford J. *Clinical lectures 1752. MS.* London: Wellcome Institute for the History of Medicine, 1752. 3. Cited in: Lawrence C. The meaning of histories. *Bull History Med,* 1992; **66**: 638–45.

23 Ehrenreich B, English D. *For her own good: 150 years of experts' advice to women.* London: Pluto Press, 1979.

24 Barrow L. Democratic epistemology: mid-ninteenth-century plebeian medicine. *Soc Soc History Med Bull* 1981; **29**: 25–9.

25 Lock M. The return of the patient as person In: Wear A. ed. *History of the doctor–patient relationship.* Euro America, Ishikayu, 1995, pp. 99–130.

26 Gibson R. *The family doctor, his life and history.* London: Allen and Unwin, 1981, p. 9.

27 Jackson S. The listening healer in the history of psychological healing. *Am J Psychiat* 1992; **149**: 1623–32.

28 Foucault M. *Discipline and punish: the birth of the prison.* London: Allen Lane, 1977, pp. 184–92.

29 Aaronovitch B. *Give it time: an experience of hospital 1928–32.* London: Deutsch, 1974, pp. 1168–9.

30 Rousseau GS. *Enlightenment borders, pre and post-modern discourses, medical, scientific.* Manchester: Manchester University Press, 1991, p. 10.

31 Gagnier M. *Subjectivities: a history of self representation in Britain, 1832–1920.* Oxford: Clarendon Press, 1991.

32 Vincent D. *Bread, knowledge and freedom: a study of nineteenth-century working-class autobiography.* London: Methuen, 1981.

33 Barnes D. *The making of a social disease: tuberculosis in nineteenth-century France.* Berkeley: University of California Press, 1995.

34 Darwin F ed. *The autobiography of Charles Darwin and selected letters.* New York: Dover, 1958, p. 40.

35 Martineau H. *Autobiography,* Volume 1. London: Virago, 1983, p. 10.

36 Bailin M. *The Sickroom in Victorian Fiction, the Art of Being Ill.* Cambridge: Cambridge University Press, 1994, p. 5.

37 McLellan FM. Literature and medicine: narratives of physical illness. *Lancet* 1997; **349**: 1618–20.

16 Nursing, narrative, and the moral imagination

P Anne Scott

Introduction

Within nursing and medicine there is currently much interest in the character, moral strategy and role enactment of health care practitioners.[1-3] Moral strategy refers to when and how we go about doing something of moral relevance; for example, when and how a patient is asked to participate in a clinical trial. Role enactment refers to the qualities an individual brings to his or her functioning in a role. These qualities are elements of a practitioner's character which cannot be reduced to aspects of the role itself.

An active moral imagination is a crucial aspect of the role enactment and moral strategy of health carers. Though it is difficult to describe precisely what moral imagination is, I suggest that for our present purposes, moral imagination is that aspect of imagination which becomes active during attempts by health care practitioners to consider what moral decisions to make; the human faculty that allows "gut-reaction" to be used and moderated into the perceptual schema, enabling a moral agent to build up multi-dimensional understandings of a situation. This faculty comprises three elemental influences: reason, gut-response and something akin to Humean fancy.[4]

I suggest it is activity of the moral imagination which at least partially allows the sensitive nurse or doctor to perceive non-verbal cues, to attend to patients sufficiently to know when someone is capable of coping with bad news, rather than merely stating such news in a cold factual way. Respecting patient autonomy is important, but given the vulnerability which illness brings, so also is considering the particular situation of an individual patient in their narrative context. If this consideration is the work of an active moral imagination,[1, 2] how might its development be supported educationally?

Murdoch's idea is that by paying attention (in Weil's sense of a just and loving gaze directed upon a person or object) properly, selflessly, one comes to see what must be done.[5] As Murdoch points out: "I can only choose within the world I can see, in the moral sense of see which implies that clear vision is a result of moral imagination and moral effort."[6] She goes on to note that: "where virtue is concerned we often apprehend more than we clearly understand and [we] grow by looking."[6]

Students of nursing and medicine are actively trained to filter out large chunks of information whilst being encouraged to focus (sometimes quite reasonably) upon physical complaints. One result of their clinical training is that the student, perhaps unconsciously, becomes aware of what can be ignored. Awareness of the psychosocial dimensions of illness sensitises one to the idea that a patient may not overtly show the effects of hospitalisation, or of being socialised into a patient mode of operation. The dehumanising effects of being ignored or depersonalised by health care staff may not be readily evident to staff whose encounters with patients may be relatively brief. However, such encounters carry moral evaluation and may harm the patient (and the staff involved for that matter). Is the health care practitioner morally responsible for interactions with patients (or other professionals), the effects of which the practitioner does not see and may not be consciously aware of?

The answer to this question must contain the phrase "it depends". It depends on whether it is reasonable to expect the practitioner to be aware of her impact on the patient, or the impact of the institution or of a certain diagnosis or treatment, upon the patient. If certain actions or attitudes would be objected to, could be found wanting, or found to cause harm to a person in ordinary social interactions, there is a good case to be made for suggesting that they will also have the same effect within a health care professional context. For example, to stick a glass tube in another person's mouth in the middle of a public bar or a shop could be described as assault. In a doctor's surgery the person is probably having her temperature taken. But to strip a person naked in a public ward (or indeed in a single room) leaving the person totally exposed is not acceptable any more than it would be acceptable to demand that a customer strip in a department store.

It would appear that many incidents similar (in the metaphorical sense) to stripping a patient naked in a public ward can become equivalent, in the mind of some health care practitioners, to taking a patient's temperature. Failure by a health care professional to listen to a patient attempting, perhaps unsuccessfully, to provide relevant information also fits into this category; as does failure to respect a person's rights or human dignity, or failure to see the patient as a person.

This type of failure results from problems with the quality of role enactment of particular practitioners; it arises from a lack of sympathy and/or empathy with the patient. Nurses (and other health care practitioners) can reasonably be expected to have imaginative sensitivities to allow and encourage feelings and attitudes of sympathy and empathy between practitioner and patient. These are essential qualities for those who describe themselves as belonging to the caring professions. Practitioners can and should be held responsible for lacking these qualities or characteristics when it causes harm to patients (or indeed to themselves as persons).

Imagination, what is its relevance?

It is not just the grosser perceptual aspects of imagination which appear to be lacking in the health care practitioner who carries on a teaching round while an old lady tries to use a bed pan.[7] In this sort of situation, it is possible to argue that it is fine tuning of the imagination that is missing. The former aspects of imagination have been discussed in depth by Hume[8] and Kant[9] and more recently by Mary Warnock; she formulates its role as one that: "bridges the gap between sensory data and intelligible thought".[10]

By "fine tuning" is meant that aspect of the imagination allowing the health professional to perceive personhood in a patient; the aspect of imagination which allows the practitioner to believe not only in the continuous existence of a particular patient, but which allows her to understand that here there exists "a person such as I". In the words of Henry James, this is the aspect of the imagination that allows one to be "finely aware and richly responsible".[11]

Moral paralysis

But are not practitioners too busy trying to get on with their jobs to have time to worry about being "finely aware and richly responsible"? Inherent in this kind of question is a criticism: too much concentration upon imagination, upon imaginative identi-fication with patients, may induce moral and professional paralysis (see Chapter 12).

However, if health care professionals are to assume ultimate responsibility for decisions having potentially profound impacts upon patients, it is vital for them to understand clearly the possible and likely implications of their decisions from within the narrative context of each patient, and not just from a medical point of view. Health care professionals have a duty to engage actively at a level which allows them to gain sufficient insight into the personal world of the patient to perceive the likely implications of certain treatment decisions for *this* particular patient. Engagement of this sort, I suggest, only comes through activating moral imagination.

The moral imagination is not a floundering at the level of uneducated emotion. It is the activity of a faculty which has been nurtured and developed within the practitioner, a faculty akin I suggest, to an intellectual virtue in Aristotle's sense of the term[12]; more particularly a faculty directly relevant to the Aristotelian virtue of phronesis (practical reason). Activity of the moral imagination is central to issues of moral strategy, role enactment and the personal characteristic of compassion; indirectly, it is therefore related to the quality of health care which the public receive.[1,2]

Without to some extent entering imaginatively into the world of the "person-who-is-the-patient", it is impossible to achieve much of the understanding upon which compassion depends. For example, it is not possible to understand the meaning or impact which breast cancer has for a 36-year-old woman unless the practitioner also learns of, and takes into consideration, for example, that this particular young woman also has five small children and an alcoholic husband. It may be suggested that whilst this extra bit of a patient's social history may well be useful to know, it is not vital. I suggest that possibly the only time in a patient's treatment that such information is *not* directly relevant to a treatment programme is in a situation of life or death, such as cardiac resuscitation. Here the only really relevant information may well be "is the heart beating?" and "is the patient breathing?" But even here, if a patient is not responding to treatment, or is not responding as well as expected, by supplying sufficient narrative for the practitioner to begin to identify imaginatively with the patient, apparently irrelevant bits of the social history feed into manage-ment considerations that can have an influence upon treatment options.[13] For all these reasons, educating the moral imagination is a crucial task for nursing and medical educators.

Non-compliance

Patients are unlikely (unless desperate) even to try to communicate adequately with practitioners who seem unable to establish a rapport with them, or who are unable to evince sympathy/ empathy or compassion. Such failures can potentially harm a patient through inappropriate treatment choices or through resulting non-compliance. These factors alone seem to provide good reasons to try to help nurses and doctors develop the capacities necessary to enable them to provide adequate humane care for their patients. But there is another relevant consideration.

If the practitioner continually fails to reach common ground with her patients in terms of developing an appreciation of what sickness means within their life and world, then not only the patient may be damaged. Murdoch suggests that we "grow by looking".[6] If one does not look, one does not learn to see. At the very least this may cause one to stagnate; at worst the practitioner is diminished by the experience. To fail to see or to understand is to be oblivious to a reality; the result is that this reality fails to enter one's world. One may stagnate behind a self-protective wall or one may be forced to channel one's energies into strengthening the wall, resulting in a shrinking of one's own humanity. Murdoch[6] and Griffin[14] suggest that such stagnation and shrinking is the result of a self-protective selfishness. A pertinent question here is: "is it selfishness or is it the painfulness of what one sometimes witnesses, that prevents one from being able to see?"

Health care practitioners may certainly witness events so painful that the desire not to look, not to see, may become overwhelming. It is precisely because health care practitioners are almost daily faced with this reality in an unadulterated, undisguised way, that their ability to look, to see, to live with and grow from such experiences is all the more necessary. For if such abilities are not fostered, desiccation of the personality, burnout, and attrition from the professions are almost inevitable scenarios.

The potential for this type of scenario to befall a practitioner provides another reason for supporting the development of practitioners' moral imagination. If health carers can imaginatively identify with patients during certain trying situations the focus of the practitioner's attention becomes directed to the patient rather than upon himself and his own particular needs (conscious or unconscious). Therefore, the practitioner's practice is patient-centred (patient-directed or patient-focused) rather than practitioner-centred; and it is this that allows an enriching and an enlarging of practitioner perspectives.

Imaginative capacity plays a very important role in both the quality of role enactment and the moral strategies which a practitioner adopts. It may also play a central role in the capacity to communicate with a patient, and in the type of person which a practitioner can become. In a useful analysis of the concept of caring in clinical practice Griffin makes some relevant remarks:

> To be able to care what must a nurse first be like? If she or he is an active participant in an important human experience, it is necessary that she is able and willing to understand the features of this situation and that the nurse is "a mind in possession of its own experience", (not everyone understands much of what happens to them) receptive too, to painful emotional questions. Part of this understanding may be built up by reflection. ... Its essential value is related to the maturity of the individual in being able to clear his mind of self-oriented concerns and obsessions. It requires some liberation from self-centredness towards awareness of another's needs. To achieve this is one of the major aims of a moral education such as many nurses and others may well not have had.[14]

Griffin's suggestion that many nurses may not receive the relevant type of moral education to allow them to perceive accurately and to understand the needs of their patients, provides much food for thought for those who are trying to teach ethics to nurses (and other health care practitioners). What are educators attempting to do in teaching ethics to health care practitioners? What should our goals be? Why is the teaching of ethics seen as a good and necessary part of the curriculum? One answer I wish to offer is that ethics is taught in an attempt to help the student become a better practitioner; better in the sense of more humane, more compassionate, more caring towards the persons who will become the practitioner's patients.

Can the moral imagination be stimulated and nurtured? Nussbaum believes that it can:

> if you really vividly experience a concrete human life, imagine what it's like to live that life, and at the same time permit yourself the full range of emotional responses to that concrete life, you will (if you have at all a good moral start) be unable to do certain things to that person. Vividness leads to tenderness, imagination to compassion.[15]

The notion of "a good moral start" developed here by Nussbaum, harks back to an Aristotelian idea of virtue,[12] and suggests that attempts to educate the moral imagination come secondary to a need to consider the character of entrants to the health care professions. This is an idea that was highlighted by the Allitt Inquiry[16] which found that attempts to stimulate, develop and educate the moral imagination will "fall on stony ground" unless imaginative capacity is viewed as an element in the developing character of the practitioner.

There is a growing school of thought which suggests that the answer to the question "can the moral imagination be stimulated and nurtured?" is a resounding "yes". The theory is that moral imagination can be stimulated and nurtured through the use of the humanities, perhaps particularly the serious reading of literature, especially fiction. Nussbaum is a persuasive contemporary supporter of this theory, and further support for this position comes from the field of literary criticism. For example, Price believes that: "Our capacity to enter imaginatively into the lives of others is a process of irreversible growth. It provides us with knowledge we can never resign and must act upon". He goes on:

> What we in turn recognise as readers is the need if we are to read with any sense at all – to feel ourselves into the moral imagination of the characters. We may shift back and forth, from inside to outside ... but we cannot begin to understand the experience the novel presents without some participation in the moral realities within which its characters live.[17]

The notion that literature can affect people's behaviour is certainly not new. In *The Republic* Plato bans poets and artists because of the potentially detrimental effects of their work upon the general population.[18] Censorship laws are based on the same premise. If some forms of literature or art can be deemed to have bad influences on people, then it seems quite reasonable to suggest that other forms of literature and art can influence people to the good, as has been argued by modern day proponents of a medical humanities literature, such as Trautmann,[19] Brody,[20] and Downie.[21]

Nussbaum, following the Aristotelian tradition, suggests that one of the more effective ways of developing and nurturing professional elements that recognise the importance of perception and emotion as well as ethics, is through the use of the novel.[15] As other authors of this book, especially Harriet Squier in Chapter 14 have pointed out, attentive reading of certain types of novel helps develop moral sensitivity and imagination by inviting the reader to go beyond her immediate experience to see the importance of the specific context; and yet to perceive also the links of common humanity binding the reader to characters in stories. It is perhaps not too difficult a step from here to developing sympathetic identification with the patients one meets in clinical practice.

This notion, of course, raises two further issues. First, if literature can stimulate the moral imagination how can we ensure that this is a positive rather than a detrimental influence on practitioner character and patient care? And second, the literature which scholars such as Nussbaum suggest may not be immediately accessible to the average medical or nursing student; how does one decide what literature to use? (See Chapters 13, 14, 21 and Appendix).

An answer to the first concern is not easy, but must be rooted in an acceptance of certain ideals of clinical practice based on the core concepts of "care" and "treatment". The answer is also directly related to identifying desirable dispositions of character in practitioners. In answer to the second problem, Nussbaum concentrates on the novel as a means of moral education. Many educators in the medical humanities use also, or exclusively, contemporary short stories, drama, and poetry (Coles[22] Trautmann[19] and Downie[21]). I suggest there are advantages in using a mixture of texts, and a mixture of media – both printed and visual. Novels and films carry the advantage of historical perspective, and lengthy descriptions of context and character. They are also good sources for developing history-taking skills in students. However, within the realities of a crowded curriculum one must be realistic in one's expectations of students. Poetry and short stories can often focus the mind sharply and effectively on an issue of concern.

Murdoch advises focusing on certain works of art, and this approach is increasingly being considered in medical and nursing education.[21] This may be very useful for those who find art accessible. However, literature has two advantages in this area: first, most of our students will have been exposed to literature until midway through their secondary education, if not afterwards. Therefore one is not working from scratch in this area. Second, literature will provide first-order and also second-order concepts with which to enrich the language and thought processes of our students. In a context where there is growing subsumption of the language of the market place into thinking, writing and policy-making about health care practice, I suggest that this is not an unimportant consideration. Language influences thought[5][23][24] and it is difficult to see how verbal thought does not affect the boundaries of imaginative activity.

Conclusion

Moral imagination is important to the quality of a practitioner's role enactment, the moral strategies adopted by a practitioner, and to a practitioner's ability to communicate with patients. The quality of care which a patient receives from a practitioner is not only to do with technical, clinical skills, but also with the practitioner's ability to listen and communicate as well as with the quality of the practitioner's role enactment and moral strategy. An active moral imagination is therefore important to the type of care which patients receive from health care practitioners.

It is further being suggested by many theorists that the moral imagination can be stimulated and nurtured through the humanities, particularly literature. If this is the case, a place should be made for the use of literature in the already crowded curriculum of medical and nursing students. This, of course, is not a new idea, however I think that an attempt to link activities of the moral imagination directly to certain aspects of patient care are a significant factor which adds weight to the demand.

This chapter is adapted and condensed from Scott PA. Imagination. *Journal of Medical Ethics* 1997; **23**: 45–50.

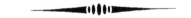

1 Scott PA. *Virtue, imaginative identification and the health care practitioner.* Unpublished PhD thesis, University of Glasgow, 1993.
2 Scott PA. Care, attention and imaginative identification in nursing practice. *J Adv Nurs* 1995; **21**: 1196–200.
3 Downie RS. *Government action and morality.* London: MacMillan, 1964.
4 Hume D. *A treatise on human nature*, 2nd edition. (Text revised by P. Nidditch.) Oxford: Clarendon Press, 1978.
5 Murdoch I. *Sovereignty of good.* London: Routledge and Kegan Paul, 1970.
6 Murdoch I. *Sovereignty of good.* London: Routledge and Kegan Paul, 1970, pp. 31–7.
7 Caplan AL. Can applied ethics be effective in health care practice and should it strive to be? *Ethics* 1983; **93**: 311–9.
8 Hume D. *An enquiry concerning the human understanding and an enquiry concerning the principles of morals.* Oxford: Clarendon Press, 1902.
9 Kant E. *A critique of judgment.* New York: Hefner, 1951.

10 Warnock M. *Imagination*. London: Faber and Faber, 1976.

11 James H. *The art of the novel*. New York: Charles Scribner and Sons, 1907.

12 Aristotle. *The nicomachean ethics*. Translated by Sir David Ross, revised by JL Ackrill and JO Urmson. Oxford: Oxford University Press, World Classics Series, 1980.

13 Kleinman A. *The illness narratives: suffering, healing and the human condition*. New York: Basic Books, 1988.

14 Griffin AP. A philosophical analysis of caring in nursing. *J Adv Nurs* 1983; **8**: 289–95.

15 Nussbaum MC. *Love's knowledge*. Oxford: Oxford University Press, 1990.

16 Clothier C (chairman). *The Allitt inquiry: independent inquiry relating to deaths and injuries on the children's ward at Grantham and Kesteven General Hospital during the period February to April 1991*. London: HMSO, 1994.

17 Price M. *Forms of life: character and moral imagination in the novel*. New Haven, CT: Yale University Press, 1983.

18 Plato. *The Republic*. Translated by Lee D. Harmondsworth: Penguin, 1974.

19 Trautmann J. *Healing arts and dialogue – medicine and literature*. Illinois: Southern Illinois University Press, 1981.

20 Brody H. *Stories of sickness*. New Haven, CT: Yale University Press, 1987.

21 Downie RS ed. *The healing arts: an Oxford illustrated anthology*. Oxford: Oxford University Press, 1994.

22 Coles R. *The call of stories: teaching and the moral imagination*. Boston: Peter Davidson, Houghton Miffin, 1989.

23 Vygotsky L. *Thought and language*. Revised and edited by Alex Kozulin. Massachusetts: MIT Press, 1986.

24 Diamond C. Losing your concepts. *Ethics* 1988; **98**: 255–77.

Dead notes: a meditation and an investigation in general practice

Brian Hurwitz

As a general practitioner (GP) in central London, I am aware of how often our practice provides a link between registered patients and their dead relatives or friends who once were also our patients. Little is known about this aspect of continuity of care. Can it survive death? What traces do deceased patients leave in general practice? How do we remember them? What networks do they leave behind?

Since the start of the practice in 1985, we have kept a death register. The intention was to use it to maintain a mortality audit, but it was mostly referred to at Christmas when writing personal notes to bereaved patients during the previous year. By permission from the health authority we retain the medical records of all patients who die while on our list. This expanding archive of dead notes is a strange reminder of past patients and of our relationship with them, their families, and survivors.

Our archive reminds me of Gogol's novel *Dead Souls*, in which a 19th-century Russian businessman, Chichikov, buys up the names of dead serfs from landowners. The more populous an estate, the greater the loan that could be secured upon it. By purchasing dead souls, an estate could become more valuable for as long as the dead names lived on in annals of official agencies. For some landowners, the names presented to Chichikov for purchase as he made his way from one estate to another meant nothing. People who had lived and worked all their lives on the land had vanished from their landowner's memory. For others, the mere mention of names evoked stories and gales of laughter; and visual memories of individuals and families, villages and rural landscapes populated with peasants, some hard working, others not, their foibles as real as when they had worked the land.

Twentieth-century GPs are the inheritors of lists of people inhabiting defined areas (practice estates). The registered list,

159

bequeathed to us by 19th-century friendly society and club practice, has been preserved by the UK National Health Service system of remuneration. Because GPs remain medical advisers to many of the surviving relatives and friends of dead patients, practices are focal points of contact with the dead. In one sense, these patients have left our registered list, but in another sense, they cannot, perhaps, ever leave.

I decided to use the practice death register to see how much the practice-GPs remembered of patients who, during the previous 9 years, had died while registered on our list. Each of the three principals in the practice responded (yes or no) to eight questions about each patient (Box).

I and another GP who had worked in the practice for 9 years examined the details (name, address, sex, age at death) of 359 patients, whereas the doctor who had worked for 4 years in the practice examined the details of a subset of 169 patients (those who had died during the 4 years she had worked in the practice). We could each remember the name of 65–69% of the patients, but could recall the face of only about half of this proportion. Aspects of personality, life story, and medical history were recalled for about a third of the patients. We each remembered being involved in the care of 31–43% of them, and we could subsequently recall caring for a relative or friend of a deceased person in 16–24% of

---

Questions asked

1 Can you recall this name?
2 Do you remember the patient's face?
3 Do you remember anything about this person's character or personality?
4 Do you remember any aspect of this patient's life story?
5 Can you remember any aspect of this patient's medical history?
6 Were you involved in the care of this patient?
7 Have you been involved in the care of a friend or relative of the patient?
8 Can you remember using your knowledge or memory of this patient after their death?

Questions 1–6 pertain to doctor memory of particular patients, whereas questions 7–8 relate to involvement with their family or social relationships and to the use of knowledge about the deceased after death.

cases, and using our knowledge and memory of the deceased in only 20% or fewer cases.

Our collective memory recalled the names of 84% of all patients; yet in only 53% could we put faces to names and recall some personality or aspect of character; in 45% of cases we would recall some aspect of patients' life stories. For 58%, some parts of a patient's medical history could be recalled, and we remembered using some aspect of our knowledge of a patient after that person's death in 28% of cases.

Complete continuity of care can be said to have taken place when to all eight questions about a patient the answer was "yes"; 20% of our patients fell into this category. However, if the answer to questions 2–6 was "no", the patient as an identifiable individual had, to all intents and purposes, vanished, though not entirely without trace. Our memory-trace of dead patients is fairly complete in 42% (questions 1–6 answered "yes"). But 35% of our dead patients had vanished from our memories: we could recall nothing at all about them other than in a few cases their names only.

The results provide an outline of the scope of our memories built up as a result of prolonged and repeated contact with individuals on our list. Though the results were not verified against any external standard, errors are likely to be self-cancelling. The exercise sensitised us to various differences between the three GPs in the practice. For example, one of us could recall the life-story in a smaller proportion of cases than could the other two, suggesting perhaps a different relationship with patient narrative, or a different tendency to retain the narrative. The doctor who had joined the practice only 4 years previously turned out to recognise the names of 100 people who had died before she had arrived in the practice – an example, perhaps, of the spill-over effects of doctor–patient relationships within the practice setting. This particular doctor misidentified only one person whom she had not known – by confusing him with another. If her error rate is typical of the three doctors, the false-positive identification rate is likely to have been less than 1%.

Studies of bereavement and mourning over the past 20 years have added greatly to our understanding of the responses by individuals and families to the death of a close family member. There have also been some good studies of mortality in general practice, and Balint and others have helped to sensitise us to our own emotional responses to individual deaths within practices.

However, no-one seems to have studied the effects on GPs of losing a population of patients over time, and little attention has been paid to the role of GPs' memory of former patients in their subsequent practice.

My exercise in GP perception involved an unstandardised questionnaire with loosely formulated questions. Nonetheless, it revealed a patchwork of continuities between past and present narratives, and it helped unlock memories of former patients, enabling us to make contact with, and to revive, inner images of our past patients. Like the landowners in *Dead Souls*, we too found ourselves laughing and reminiscing about people we had known and cared for. We have gained, in the process, a better understanding of the extent to which we carry with us, in fragmented form, experiences and awareness of dead patients.

Certain deaths had been more tragic and personally sad to us than others. We felt uncomfortable about patients who had apparently vanished from our collective memory. We were more likely to have forgotten patients who had died after moving into residential accommodation, and this engendered a sense of guilt. But the exercise as a whole has brought us closer to a tapestry of memories: of impressions, predicaments, jokes, personal imprints, traces, gifts, words, images, pain, successes, guilt, and failures, which form part of the unfolding narrative of general practice.

John Berger has observed that GPs occupy, as "the familiar of death", the position of living intermediaries between the community and its "multitudinous dead". Recognising the extent and limitations of our recollections has helped balance our thinking and feeling in this area of practice.

Acknowledgments

I thank Berry Beaumont and Imogen Bloor, my partners at 2 Mitchison Road Practice, London N1, UK, for agreeing to take part in this study, and for allowing me to report on our experiences in practice during our first 9 years of partnership. I also thank Ruth Richardson for numerous discussions of the ideas developed here, and for commenting upon the paper. Further tabulated details of the results of this study are available from the author.

This chapter was originally published in *The Lancet* 1988; **351**: 593–4. Reproduced here by permission.

Understanding narrative in health care

17 Stories we hear and stories we tell . . . analysing talk in clinical practice

Glyn Elwyn and Richard Gwyn

Even at its scientific best, medicine is always a social act.[1]

For all the science which underpins clinical practice, we make sense of the world around us, practitioners as much as patients, by way of stories.[2][3] Even the most evidence-crazed doctors have to translate their perception of "biostatistical truths" into accounts which make sense to others. Yet it is only in the last 40 years or so that attention has been given to the forms of talk that occur between clinicians and patients, to the stories exchanged. Studies of the consultation process in medicine, which have largely taken place in primary care, have focused on the structure of the meeting[4] and on the phases[5] which can be described from greeting to closure. Differing communication styles have been identified[6] and it has been noted that, more often than not, despite a clear need to adapt to circumstances, doctors have very fixed ways of talking with patients. The concepts of "doctor" or "patient" centredness are described[7] and measured;[8] concepts which are undoubtedly having a profound influence on professional practice.[9] These observations have led in turn to an ongoing exploration of the effect that communication styles have on both patient satisfaction levels and clinical outcomes.[10]

It could be argued, however,[11] that there is much more depth to be explored within the discourse that occurs between a clinician and a patient, and that the tools normally employed – even the semi-quantitative methods of analysing patient-centredness – cannot be used to examine the layers of meanings which lie within the text of medical exchanges. Selected and trained as if they were being prepared to be "scientists", doctors are seldom interested in

165

these issues and it is not easy to find a way into the methods from other disciplines which could uncover the subtle and intricate interactions that take place within a clinical interview. Paradoxically, the need to understand the decision-making processes which occur within the "black box" of the consultation is increasing. The dual forces of economics and evidence-based medicine are defining the limits of clinical freedom, and the equal, but sometimes opposing, pressures of patient choice and increasing access to information are raising the stakes. Could the micro-analysis of talk inform the essence of medical practice; define principles for effective communication; attach meanings to a patient's individual story as well as help doctors share ideas about fears and hopes for the future – in medical-speak, communicate "risks and benefits"?[12] By deconstructing a piece of dialogue, down to the last breath, we hope to illustrate the value of learning to listen, in great detail, to the stories we hear.

Illnesses, quite apart from their biological existence, are socially constructed events, reproduced and perpetuated through talk, and most specifically, through narratives, which are the most basic of discourse units.[13] Doctors commonly refer to the "course of an illness" and regard this "course" (a metaphor of journey) as a sequential experience which lends itself naturally to a linear narrative form. The basic task of clinical training is to "take" and "give" histories: and it is through the hearing and telling of stories that human beings have always come to understand their experiences.[14][15] According to one commentator, this narrative frame is as valid for clinicians as it is for the victims of illness. Despite doctors' attempts to retain an "objective" presentation of "the facts", they were found frequently to interrupt seminars with accounts that began with phrases such as "there was this one guy".[2] Recent developments in cognitive science indicate a growing awareness of the central role that narratives play in the way that people make meanings,[16] and it has even been suggested that human grammars arose out of a proto-linguistic need to narrate.[17] Frequently, we come across narratives embedded in the fabric of a wider discourse – an 'interview' or 'conversation' – and it is with this in mind that we approach the discipline of discourse analysis, a form of textual microscopy, which will be employed as the analytical framework of this chapter.

Essentially discourse analysis is the study of language in context.[18][19] Studies of how doctors talk to patients at outpatient clinics,[20] how health visitors discuss issues with their clients[21] and how HIV counsellors convey information and advice[22] are examples where these techniques have revealed valuable but previously hidden patterns and perspectives. Discourse analysis, as practised here, has roots in linguistics, sociology and psychology, but despite these disparate origins it is really no more than the examination of processes of naturally occurring talk. By focusing on its organisation and sequences, we are able to discern the *rhetorical* organisation of everyday talk: how, for instance, is one version of events selected over and above any other; how is a familiar reality described in language in such a way as to lend it normative and unquestionable authority? On a broader front, discourse analysis is "concerned with examining discourse (whether spoken or written) to see how cognitive issues of knowledge and belief, fact and error, truth and explanation are conceived and expressed".[18] The one essential thing to remember about "doing" discourse analysis is that we stick to the text, which in many cases, like the following extract, is a piece of talk, a consultation between a general practitioner and a patient.

The patient is a woman, aged 52, visiting an inner-city practice. Because she has an urgent problem she has been unable to see her "usual" doctor and has to consult with a practitioner she has not met before. She begins with a torrent of symptoms: puffy eyes and legs; burning urine; going backwards and forwards to the toilet; pain in the back and a sore throat. Whilst her story emerges the doctor examines the urine sample she has given to him. He diagnoses a "water infection" (she gets recurrent urine infections) and asks the patient if she is allergic to any antibiotics. She responds with a sigh and the words: "I feel *terrible*". "Terrible" can mean so much, and so little. In the English of South Wales it is employed, as one clinician has remarked, as a standard descriptive term for almost any condition.[15] At this point the consultation might well have terminated with a prescription. But then the patient lets out a cough. Nothing extravagant. Just a little cough.

Let's turn then to the transcript and employ the techniques of discourse analysis at first hand. The aim is to reproduce the dialogue down to the last "um". It contains symbols which can seem at first a bit off-putting. Interruptions, pauses, overlapping speech and intonations are all signified. The detail of the transcription is an essential part of doing discourse analysis: we need to gain access to the precise dynamics of the interaction. Brackets containing a stop (.) indicate a pause of less than 2 seconds. Numerals in round brackets indicate the length in seconds of other pauses. Square brackets [ ] contain relevant contextual information, italicised square brackets *[.]* describe a non-verbal utterance. The symbol [in between lines of dialogue, indicates overlapping speech. Under<u>lin</u>ing signifies emphasis and an equal sign = means that the phrase is contiguous with the preceding phrase without pause. A colon : indicates elongation of the preceding sound, as in *uh:*. We are 2 minutes 30 seconds into a consultation which lasts 6 minutes 45 seconds in total. The extract which follows lasts 2 minutes:

047	D	. . I'm going to give you something called Augmentin
048		it's a little white <u>bull</u>et (.)
049		if you take them three times a day (.)
		[
050	P	mhm
051	D	and we'll see if it helps you
052	P	okay that's lovely *[coughs briefly]*
053	D	anything else?
054		(.)
055	P	uh (.) dya dya oh is it Dyazide? (.)
056		the (.) water tablets I'm on?
057	D	you take those regularly?
058	P	yeah <u>every</u> day (.)
059		now I always take them in the <u>morn</u>ing but (.)
060		would it be all right to take them in the <u>night</u>? (.)
061		you know because oh *[sighing]*
062		it drives me mad you know
063		cos I (.) pass water <u>so</u> much =
064	D	= course you do =
065	P	= and as I say if I'm on holiday I think well
066		I don't want to be running into the toilet all the time
067	D	why are you taking (.) water tablets?
068	P	because I'm on HRT?
069	D	oh yeah =
070	P	= um (.) Clif Clif Cilafin is it? well I've got enough of those (.)
		[
071	D	mmm: mm
072	P	but I wanted the er Seroxat
073		the antidepressant tablets please
074	D	you <u>take</u> those do you?
075	P	yeah
076	D	how long have you been taking those?
077	P	(.) uh: well my son was killed (2.0) 5 years ago (2.0)
078		just after that then (.) 3 months after (.)
079		my (.) <u>grand</u>daughter

080		3 month old twin granddaughter died of meningitis (.)
081		then in the January (.) my son in law got uh
082		died of a heart complaint
083		22 so I re<u>fused</u> to take anything you know
084		but <u>then</u> (.) doctor Y <u>insisted</u> (.)
085		and I <u>have</u> found them and I started <u>work</u>
086		after 30 years I'm a re<u>cep</u>tionist at the um
087		[names famous Welsh institution] (.)
088		and I have <u>really</u> found that <u>that</u> has (.)
089		been <u>more</u> of a help to me (.) *[breathes heavily]*
090		but doctor Y said she <u>still</u> wanted me to take those antidepressants
091		but <u>I</u> was thinking (.) would I be able to take <u>one</u> one day
092		leave one off the next day
093		to try and (.) would you know
094		would that be all right do you think or?
095	D	do you want to do that?

When the doctor completes prescribing (047–051), the patient responds with "okay that's lovely" (052), and what might best be described as a discreet cough. The cough, in these circumstances, apparently functions as a *discourse marker* signalling the speaker's wish *not* to terminate the interaction.[23] The doctor's next utterance "anything else" is characteristic of doctors' pre-closing moves in medical interactions[24] and suggests that the consultation might be closed here, but leaves such closure to the patient. The patient (P) is in a position to enable the doctor (D) to proceed to closing, or herself to shift to a new topic. She opts to respond (055), after a false start, first with a pause, then a request for "water tablets." The pause here indicates that there is to be a new topic, but it precludes any accusation of indecent haste, suggesting that the patient does not wish to be perceived simply as itemising a shopping list. The ritual of correct timing is necessary in order to maintain the necessary gravity accorded to the ceremony of consultation and prescription. Although the pause lasts less than 2 seconds, its significance should not therefore be underestimated.

While seeming to struggle with the brand name, P effectively foregrounds the new topic of her "water tablets", phrasing the statement/question with a high rising tone: "is it Dyazide? (.) the (.) water tablets I'm on?" (055–056). A high rising tone is a vernacular feature that involves a rising intonation pattern on

169

utterances which *function* as statements.[25] The high rising tone often serves as a facilitative device, inviting confirmation. The doctor's response is one of apparent puzzlement: "you take those regularly?" (057), in which the word "regularly" acts as a qualifier which begs the more relevant question of why the patient takes them at all. Once the patient has completed her explanation (065–066), the doctor asks the question "why are you taking water tablets?" (067), to which the answer ("because I'm on HRT") is again delivered with a high rising tone, which seems either to indicate uncertainty as to the correctness of this response or else questions the relevance of the doctor's question. As an answer to D's question, however, it is of no help, since it does not provide a satisfactory biomedical reason. The doctor *hedges* the explanation[25] ("oh yeah") *without* however committing himself in any way to an acceptance of P's given explanation. But already, P is moving on to the next topic. She dismisses the water tablet topic while D is still mulling it over – a prolonged "mmm:" (071) – and proceeds (072–073): "I wanted the er Seroxat the antidepressant tablets please".

The use of the past tense ("I wanted") for a present tense request serves as a means by which the speaker removes herself from the here and now, a common feature of "negative politeness".[26] This is consistent with a reluctance to be perceived as too pushy or demanding, and consolidated by the "please" at the end of the utterance. The doctor's response this time indicates a less restrained surprise: "you *take* those do you?" Having just queried (067) P on her use of diuretics, and apparently unconvinced ("mmm:", 071) by her explanation, D might be reluctant to bluntly ask P about the source of her depression, but at the same time the seemingly unrelated sequence of her taking water tablets, HRT, and her call for antidepressants, demands rather more substantiation. Moreover, perhaps, the doctor needs to assert his professional role as custodian of the drugs cabinet. P replies to the question ("you take those do you?", the slight but unexpected emphasis on "take" indicating D's momentary confoundedness) with a simple "yeah" (075), and D follows up with a question formulated out of professional concern and framed in linear time: "how long have you been taking those?"

There is a pause, a false start again (uh:), and then P chooses to respond not in linear time, but in event time: "well my son was killed" (077) – the event which for her began the sequence of events which culminated in her being prescribed antidepressants on a regular basis. These opening phrases are interspersed by lengthy pauses:

> (.) uh: well my son was killed (2.0) 5 years ago (2.0).

Linear time (5 years) is only relevant in relation to event time (her son's death). On this subject, Mishler[11] has made the famous distinction between the "voice of medicine" and the "voice of the lifeworld". He cites a consultation between a general practitioner and a young woman who is abusing alcohol.

D: . . . .
. . . . . How long have you been drinking that heavily?
P: . . . . Since I've been married.
D: . . . . .
. . . . How long is that?
P: (giggle) Four years. (giggle)

Mishler, dismissing the importance of a biomedical time frame for clinical judgments, argues that the practitioner, by insisting on a 'real' time scale (4 years) over a more meaningful, personal one, subordinates the voice of the lifeworld to the voice of medicine. The comparison with our example is clear, but the doctor in our case does *not* interrupt the patient, allows her time to pause, to tell her story. A first pause leaves D discursive space to come in if he wishes, but he does not. By not interfering D allows the voice of the lifeworld to take precedence (i.e. life-meaning comes before time-meaning) but by so doing he gives P the opportunity to fill in the kinds of linear detail which she thinks might be relevant, and which she immediately does anyway ("5 years ago").

More important to our argument is the means by which this introduction of biographical detail helps establish a narrative basis to the patient's depression and thus legitimises her continued use of antidepressants. The account, with its litany of deaths, provides the general practitioner with an idea of this patient's "sustaining fiction",[27] of the explanatory causes which underlie her story. We are all continuously involved in the process of adding new stories to the sustaining fictions of our own biographies, of accounting for "how things are". The whole biographical process is a narrative-making endeavour. Stories are renewed, reconstructed or abandoned, but are always central to the individual's presentation of self and sense of personal identity. So when we examine this fragment's precise formulation we find (077) that P's son did not simply "die". Rather, the doctor is being asked to take in that P's son was "killed", that is, suffered death as the victim of a particular agent or set of circumstances. There is implicit in the pauses here the opportunity for D to request *how* her son came to be killed, an opportunity that he chooses not to take. However the pauses do act as a rhetorical device, allowing for the gravity of her loss to sink in, and accounting for the prescribed drugs. But that is not all. Seeing that D does not request further information about the circumstances of her son's death (a request which, in any case, would be highly threatening to both parties), P then enumerates two other losses in her family; the death of a baby granddaughter from meningitis, and the loss of a son-in-law from a heart complaint. The fact that the causes of death and the ages of the dead are enumerated in both these other cases only draws attention back to the lack of explanation regarding the killing of her son.

By emphasising the extent of her losses within a short space of time, P is avoiding the possibility of being categorised as somebody requesting antidepressants without good cause. Hanging over every patient is the potential accusation of malingering,[28] resulting in the obligation to prove that the malady is not contrived and to express a wish to get well, a position reinforced by this patient's immediate assurance that she "refused to take anything" (083) (i.e. any drugs). Indeed, as she recounts, it was only at her doctor's instigation (doctor Y insisted) that she began taking antidepressants at all. Having done so, she "started work after 30 years", again justifying the sick role by a demonstrable commitment to society and the work ethic. She names the well-known institution where she works with a degree of pride. Moreover, she insists that it was her doctor who "wanted her" to take the tablets (reinforcing her own passivity in this decision, despite their effectiveness) – and then (as if further evidence of her good intentions were needed) she states her wish to reduce the doses, thus maintaining her contractual responsibilities to recovery. This wish to lower the dosage is shown as her choice, unaided (indeed hindered) by her practitioner ("doctor Y said she still wanted me to take those antidepressants"), strengthening the representation of herself as a responsible member of society, one who understands and respects the dangers of prescribed drugs, a piece of self-imaging that she repeats a few lines further on: "I wouldn't like the thought of being on them for ever" (079–082).

P is now searching for a strategy to reduce or stop her use of antidepressants, and has asked D outright whether it is all right to take her tablets every other day. For the doctor, the narrative has appeared out of the blue. He records:

One second I had been prescribing Dyazide and oestrogens, the next I'm following the death processions of her son, granddaughter and son-in-law. Added to which she neatly telescopes a declaration that she's ready now to move on. Would that be all right? To withdraw from medication. To effectively contradict my partner. To participate in a shared decision about the end of grief, about a symbolic farewell to a son, killed 5 years ago. I hadn't expected this. I attempted to give her autonomy over her decision, yet hoping not to abandon her,[29] offering a firm steer that firstly it would be safe to withdraw and secondly that she was going about it in the correct way. This wasn't enough it seemed. She wanted to know what I thought about the decision.[30] How could I tell her that I didn't know? That if I had lost a son I can't imagine surviving at all, never mind coming off tablets. I suppose my hunch was that she wanted to try it out, so I went along with that, using posture more than words.

How then does discourse analysis help doctors to understand the inner workings of a consultation? The example provided, we contend, illustrates much that deserves attention. It reveals intricate communication strategies, informs us how patients construct their roles within consultations and opens up a new way of "listening" to the signals which so often pass by unnoticed: gets us that step nearer to reconstructing "the imaginative universe in which human acts are signs".[31] Mishler,[11] reviewing medical interview research, objects to mere code-category assessments, arguing for a more eclectic approach, using detailed textual assessment. As more studies demonstrate that patients' "perceptions" of what happens within consultations is probably more valid than measures based on coding-structures[32-34] and that "finding common ground" is more a *perceived* event than a quantifiable finding,[34] those who are interested in this field need methods which start illuminating the subtext, the "white space" which signifies thoughts, disagreements, distress and indecisions. The evidence emerging[34 35] that "participating" in decisions significantly reduces subsequent use of laboratory and referral services indicates the critical, but almost neglected, part that patient–doctor interaction plays in the use of health resources.

We may also have to go beyond the consultation itself to the perceived messages which patients take away with them into their own context – into the longitudinal discourse of their own lives.[36] We believe that such analysis helps provide insight into various dimensions of the consultation that would otherwise have been overlooked. As such, it provides an incisive tool for research and, in certain cases, for training, in many areas of clinical practice.[37] By being aware of certain signalling practices and discourse markers in the patient's talk, general practitioners might be able to listen more constructively to their patients' stories[38] and allow a more "democratic arrangement of voices".[39] Added to which, lest we forget, for countless patients, it is the telling of their stories that helps to make them well.

————••◆••————

1 Davidoff F. *Who has seen a blood sugar?* Philadelphia: ACP, 1996.
2 Hunter KM. *Doctors' Stories.* Princeton: Princeton University Press, 1991.
3 Brody H. *Stories of Sickness.* New Haven: Yale University Press, 1987.
4 Byrne PS and Long BEL. *Doctors talking to patients.* London: HMSO, 1976.
5 Pendleton D, Schofield T, Tate P, Havelock P. *The consultation: an approach to learning and teaching.* Oxford: Oxford University Press, 1984.
6 Roter DL, Hall JA. *Doctors talking with patients, patients talking with doctors.* Dover, MA: Auburn House, 1992.
7 Levenstein JH. The patient-centred general practice consultation. *South African Family Practice* 1984; **5**: 276–82.
8 Stewart M, Brown JB, Weston WW *et al. Patient Centred Medicine: Transforming the Clinical Method.* Thousand Oaks, CA: Sage Publications, 1995.
9 Laine C, Davidoff F. Patient-centred medicine: a professional evolution. *J Am Med Assoc* 1996; **275**: 152–6.
10 Kinnersley P. *The patient-centredness of consultations and the relationship to outcomes in primary care.* Unpublished MD thesis, University of Bristol, 1997.
11 Mishler E. *The Discourse of Medicine: Dialectics of Medical Interviews.* Norwood, NJ: Ablex, 1984.
12 Calman KC, Royston GHD. Risk language and dialectics. *Br Med J* 1997; **315**: 939–42.
13 Linde C. *Life stories: the creation of coherence.* New York: OUP, 1993.
14 Churchill L, Churchill S. Storytelling in medical arenas: the art of self-determination. Lit Med 1982; **1**: 73–9.
15 Gwyn R. *The Voicing of Illness: narrative and metaphor in personal illness accounts.* Unpublished PhD thesis, University of Wales: Cardiff, 1997.
16 Edwards D. *Discourse and Cognition.* London: Sage, 1997.
17 Bruner J. *Acts of Meaning.* Cambridge, MA: Harvard University Press, 1990.
18 Edwards D, Potter J. *Discursive Psychology.* London: Sage, 1992.
19 Potter J, Wetherell M. *Discourse and social psychology.* London: Sage, 1987.
20 Wodak R. *Disorders of Discourse.* London: Longman, 1996.
21 Drew P, Heritage J eds. *Analyzing Talk at Work.* Cambridge: Cambridge University Press, 1992.
22 Silverman D. *Discourses of Counselling.* London: Sage, 1997.
23 Coupland J, Robinson J, Coupland N. Frame negotiation in doctor–elderly patient consultations. *Discourse Soc* 1994; **5**(1): 89–124.
24 Coulthard RM, Ashby MC. A linguistic description of doctor–patient interviews. In: Wadsworth M, Robinson D eds. *Studies in everyday medical life.* London: Martin Robinson, 1976.
25 Holmes J. *An introduction to sociolinguistics.* London: Longman, 1992.
26 Brown P, Levinson SC. *Politeness: some universals in language usage.* Cambridge: Cambridge University Press, 1978.
27 Hillman J. *Healing Fiction.* Woodstock, CT: Spring Publications, 1983.
28 Parson T. *The Social System.* Glencoe: The Free Press, 1951.

29 Quill TE, Cassel CK. Nonabandonment: a central obligation for physicians. *Ann Intern Med* 1995; **122**: 368–74.
30 Quill TE, Brody H. Physician recommendations and patient autonomy: Finding a balance between physician power and patient choice. *Ann Intern Med*, 1996; **125**: 763–9.
31 Geertz C. *The interpretation of cultures.* New York: Basic Books, 1973.
32 Tuckett D, Boulton M, Olson I, Williams A. *Meetings between experts: an approach to sharing ideas in medical consultations.* London: Tavistock Publications, 1985.
33 Margalith I, Shapiro A. Anxiety and patient participation in clinical decision-making: the case of patients with ureteral calculi. *Soc Sci Med* 1997; **45**: 419–27.
34 Stewart M, Brown JB, Donner A, McWhinney IR, Oates J *et al. The impact of patient-centred care on patient outcomes in family therapy.* London, Ontario: Centre for Studies in Family Medicine, University of Western Ontario, 1997.
35 Redelmeier DA, Molin JP, Tibshirani RJ. A randomised trial of compassionate care for the homeless in an emergency department. *Lancet* 1995; **345**: 1131–4.
36 Charles C, Gafni A, Whelan T. Shared decision-making in the medical encounter: what does it mean? (Or it takes at least two to tango). *Soc Sci Med* 1997; **44**: 681–92.
37 Nessa J, Malterud K. Discourse analysis in general practice: a sociolinguistic approach. *Fam Pract* 1990; 7: 77–83.
38 Kleinman A. *The illness narratives.* New York: Basic Books, 1988.
39 Silverman D. *Communication and medical practice: social relations and the clinic.* Bristol: Sage Publications, 1987.

18 Narrative in psychotherapy

Jeremy Holmes

> It still strikes me as strange that the case histories I write should read like short stories and that, as one might say, they lack the serious stamp of science. I must console myself with the reflection that the nature of the subject is evidently responsible for this, rather than any preference of my own.[1]

As my opening quotation implies, Freud was troubled by the discrepancy between the novelistic quality of psychoanalytic discourse as it emerged in his writings, and his wish to establish psychoanalysis as a science. But for him there was no fundamental difficulty in reconciling these two facets of his project. He viewed the unconscious rather in the way that today's neuroimaging experts see the brain – an organ that is inaccessible and in many ways mysterious but which, given the right technology, can be clearly illuminated and if necessary manipulated. For him, that technology was the psychoanalytic method: free association, dream interpretation, the analysis of transference. His basic model remained that of dream interpretation which he devised at the outset of psychoanalysis. The patient brings to treatment an incomplete and incomprehensible story – whether of a dream or a symptom. By reconstructing the underlying *unconscious* story, psychoanalysis fills in the missing gaps and so rearranges the confusion until it forms a coherent narrative. Like a good detective, the culprit – usually unconscious infantile wishes – is finally identified and brought to book.

In the ensuing century, Freud's confidence in the scientific status of psychoanalysis has been challenged in many ways. Eschewing the notion of the unconscious, behaviourism offered itself as a scientific alternative to the romanticism of psychoanalysis. Evidence and evaluation were built into this psychological, as opposed to psychoanalytic, approach. The 1970s and 80s saw a vast amount of research devoted to the question of the effectiveness or otherwise of psychotherapy. The conclusion was a resounding endorsement of psychotherapy as a treatment for psychological disorders.

However, many new questions were thrown up by this research, especially as, on the whole, no one modality of psychotherapy was shown to be more effective than any other.

This finding links in with the psychoanalytic realisation that, for any given patient, there appears to be no unique psychoanalytic narrative. A Kleinian, or a Kohutian, or Kernbergian, or an interpersonal or a contemporary Freudian or a Lacanian reading of the patient will each produce a significantly different story. There is of course "common ground" between the different psychoanalytic discourses,[2] but this is still very different to the situation in the physical sciences, where, in general, there is little dispute about what constitute the "facts" of the situation, even if there may be competing theories about how best to explain them.

Further, it is clear that the "material" of psychoanalysis does not arise solely from the patient and the story she tells; it is a joint product of analyst and patient, and the theories espoused by the former have a major influence on the shape and meaning of the treatment.

This debate within psychoanalysis touches on a wider philosophical discussion about the role of narrative in everyday life, in which Alisdair Macintyre[3] and Jerome Bruner[4] are leading exponents. For Macintyre personhood and narrative are inseparable. Motives are aims within an historical context. Actions can only be understood within the context of an implicit history or story: "stories are lived before they are told". In trying to understand our own and others' behaviour we seek an underlying story which will explain their actions in this reading, psychoanalysis is an elaboration of this common-sense folk psychology. Freud's discovery was that seemingly incomprehensible symptoms could be explained if agency was attributable to unconscious motivation – a "second reality".[5]

Jerome Bruner[4] is similarly concerned to give narrative its full philosophical due. He argues that there are two kinds of approaches to truth:

> A good story and a well-formed argument are different natural kinds. Both can be used as a means for convincing another. Yet what they convince of is fundamentally different: arguments convince of their truth, stories of their lifelikeness. The one verifies by eventual appeal to procedures for establishing formal and empirical truth. The other establishes its truth by verisimilitude.

Critics of psychotherapy might argue that this is a concession that the stories elaborated in psychotherapy can lay no more claim to the truth than can myths or fairy stories. Bruner's response, I believe, would be that there is truth in myths and fairy stories – emotional truth rather than factual truth, which can be judged, not by scientific standards, but by such tests as whether the story rings true, feels right, is satisfying, coherent, or touches the listener emotionally.

The criteria of a "good story" certainly apply to psychotherapy. A psychotherapist is constantly using her intuition to evaluate the patient's narrative, asking herself if it makes sense or hangs together, questioning aspects that don't quite fit, probing clichés or phrases and well-worn narratives for what might lie beneath. The quest is always for a more elaborated, all-embracing, spontaneous, individualised, flexible story that encompasses a greater range of experience.

This evaluative activity, akin to Spence's[6] view of therapy as a branch of aesthetics, is part of the "art" of psychotherapy. But can there also be a science of narrative, including one which would encompass the narrative aspects of psychotherapy?

The main drawback of radical narrativism is the implication that a psychotherapeutic narrative is no more or less likely to be true than any other account of the patient's distress, whether religious, narrowly "organic" in the psychiatric sense, or delusional. The hermeneutic turn in psychotherapy threatens to cut psychotherapy off from aspects of science – especially from evolutionary biology and developmental psychology – where dialogue is both necessary and possible. I shall argue therefore for a *partial* narrativism, a position which includes both scientific and hermeneutic elements. While the therapeutic effect of psychotherapy may be seen as essentially narrative based, this can be buttressed by science as outcomes and techniques are evaluated using statistical methods, just as historians use carbon dating and statistics to support their search for accurate historical narrative. In addition, the findings of attachment research, which brings together the "art" of psycho-analysis with the "science" of ethology, suggests ways in which aspects of narrative in adult life can be connected with observable developmental experience in childhood.

The contribution of attachment research

While the immediate goal of psychotherapy may be to remove symptoms, behind that lies a set of more general and more ambitious objectives – to help an individual to flourish, to foster wellbeing, and so on. These can be seen in terms of the development of a strengthened and more versatile set of selves, for example: a more secure self, a more creative self, a more coping self, a more resilient self, a more autonomous self, a self with a greater capacity for intimacy. In contrast with the Cartesian *cognito,* narrative theory (as of MacIntyre) sees the "I" not as a fixed and pre-existing entity, but as an autobiographical self, formed out of the interplay between agency and contingency, needing to be "told" to another – or storied before it can come into being.[7] The telling of a self implies a built-in dialogical structure. There is always an Other to whom the Self is telling his or her story, even if in adults this takes the form of an internal dialogue.

What are the origins of this "self-story"? How do we begin to learn about ourselves and our feelings? For psychoanalysts Winnicott's notion of maternal *mirroring* provides a model both of normal development, and of the possible role of therapy. When the mother looks at the baby, according to Winnicott,[8] "*what she looks like* [to the baby] *is related to what she* [the mother] *sees there*". This clinical insight has recently been expanded by Gergely and Watson[9] who suggest that an attuned mother helps her infant identify feelings by mirroring behaviour that has two characteristics. First, the mother's facial expressions of emotion are *marked* by exaggeration, so that the child can see that they are "pretend", not real. Second, they are *contingent* on the child's feelings, so that they arise only when he or she appears to be experiencing a particular emotion, a response which in itself has a soothing function. Here we see the beginnings of a possible representation of, or story about, the self and its feelings. Marking is related to the highlighting, figure-groundedness of narrative. It is as though the mother is saying "This is you, and your feelings that you are looking at, not me". Contingency is linked with the way in which, unlike "real life", stories hang together in a coherent way, since the mother makes sure that her responses always follow the baby's lead with, as it were, a beginning, middle, and end, in contrast to the unstructured flow of "normal" responsiveness.

Gergely and Watson's speculations are based on the three decades of research on infant–mother interaction arising from Bowlby's attachment theory.[10] Recent developments in attachment research have begun to link this understanding of early life with clinical narrative in adults. The *way* we tell stories reflects our fundamental stance towards the world. The development of the

Adult Attachment Interview (AAI) by Mary Main and her colleagues[11] in the mid-1980s provided a scientific tool which was sophisticated enough to pick up some of the subtleties of the narratives which are the stuff of clinical reality.

As a psychometric instrument, the AAI is original in that its scoring system is based not so much on content as on the form and structure of the subject's *narrative* style. Narratives are classified into one of four categories: secure-autonomous, insecure-dismissive, insecure-enmeshed, and disorganised (or unresolved). The key quality of *secure-autonomous* narratives is coherence: the subject is able to speak logically and concisely about her past and its vicissitudes, however problematic these may have been. *Insecure-dismissive* narratives (equivalent to avoidant attachment styles) are unelaborated and unrevealing: the subject may state that she has no memories of her childhood before the age of 11, or that her parents were "brilliant", without being able to amplify or produce relevant examples. By contrast, in *insecure-enmeshed* narratives (equivalent to ambivalent attachment styles) the subject appears bogged down in her history, telling rambling and inconclusive stories as though past pain was still alive today. The *unresolved* category is rated separately, coexisting with the others, and referring to points in a narrative where the logical flow is interrupted, broken, or disjointed. Main suggests that these narrative fractures may represent the emergence of previously repressed traumatic memories, and may be related clinically to dissociative states.

The findings of attachment research suggest that there may be objective criteria coherence – succinctness, relevance, etc. – by which to evaluate the "verisimilitude" of a clinical narrative. It also points to powerful links between the "narrative truth" of the clinical situation and the "historical truth" of the patient's actual biography, since longitudinal studies have established the connections between secure-autonomous narratives as told by adolescents, and secure attachment as measured in infancy; similarly, children who are insecurely attached tend, when grown up, to adopt a dismissive or enmeshed narrative style.

Implications for psychotherapy

What is the relevance of this for therapeutic practice? Patients seek help in a state of uncertainty and confusion. Something is "wrong", but they do not know what this is, or what to do about it. Footsteps may have to be retraced: a story is needed which will both explain how they arrived where they are and point the way forward. Psychotherapy, like art, "holds a mirror up to nature". The patient learns to put his or her feelings into words; these are then "reflected back" by the therapist (marking); the patient then rechecks this reflection for its congruence/contingency/verisimilitude – whether it "feels right"; finally a representation, or story is formed.

The narrative approach within psychoanalysis described in the first section of this chapter has, however, not gone unchallenged. The most powerful critique of narrative has come from Lacan and his followers. Lacan[12] was consistently and implacably anti-narrative. For him the stories we tell about our lives are unavoidably alienated from the reality of experience, defensive compensations for our helplessness in the fact of an imposed linguistic and societal order symbolised by the *no(m) du pere* – the paternal prohibition and "naming" that takes us away from the primeval maternal experience, that is beyond words and stories.

This uncompromising view has to be seen in the context of Lacan's reaction to American ego-psychology which he saw as a betrayal of the radicalism of the psychoanalytic message. If we turn, as Bollas[13] has done, to Freud's original model of dream interpretation, an integration of the narrative with Lacan's anti-narrative critique becomes possible. Bollas describes a cycle in which raw unnarrativised experience is assembled each night in the form of "day's residues" into a dream narrative, and then "cracked up" each morning as the dream is dispersed and a further set of fresh experiences presents themselves. Bollas[13] takes this as a general paradigm for the activity of the unconscious which he sees as continuously fashioning lived life into stories, and then dismantling and dispersing those stories in the light of further experience. Unlike the conscious stories that we tell ourselves, dreams are stories shaped by the unconscious. The meaning of the dream or of the self-narrative is a synthesis, reflecting both the rules of narrative logic of the conscious mind, and the shaping influence of unconscious emotional responsiveness and need. In therapy the patient learns to build up a "story-telling function" which takes experience from "below", and in the light of overall meanings "from above" (which can be seen as themselves stored or condensed stories) supplied by the therapist, fashions a new narrative about her self and her world.

Narrative as a therapeutic technique

How does the psychotherapist function as an "assistant auto-biographer"?

The first task of the therapist is to assist the patient to tell her story. The starting point will be some form of distress: desires have been thwarted, or hopes dashed. The attachment research outlined above suggests that secure attachment is marked by coherent stories that convince and hang together, where detail and overall plot are congruent, and where the teller is not so detached that affect is absent, is not dissociated from the content of her story, nor so overwhelmed that her feelings flow formlessly into every crevice of the dialogue. Insecure attachment, by contrast, is characterised either by stories that are over-elaborated and enmeshed (unmarked), or by dismissive poorly fleshed-out accounts that lack contingency testing. In one it is barely possible to discern a coherent story at all; in the other the story is so schematic or vague that it lacks the detail upon which verisimilitude depends.

Starting with the assessment interview, the therapist will use her narrative competence to help the patient shape the story into a more coherent pattern. With an enmeshed patient the therapist will introduce frequent "shaping" remarks or punctuations such as "We'll come back to what happened to you as a child in a minute; first let's hear more about what is troubling you right now ..." Note the "We'll; Let's" construction in which therapist and patient are brought into a unitary position as joint students of the story. This is the beginnings of objectification, but also a model for an internal observing ego (or self-reflexive self) that can listen to and modulate feelings. Shaping a story is the narrative version of the modulation and responsiveness of the security-transmitting care-giver.

With a dismissive patient the therapist will elicit narrative in a different way, always searching for detailed images, memories and examples that bring perfunctory stories to life. "What was your mother like?"; "Can you remember an incident that illustrates that?"; "When did you first start to feel so miserable?"; "When you say you feel depressed, what does that feel like?"; "Whereabouts in your body do you experience your unhappiness?"

In both cases, the therapist offers intermittent summarising or marking remarks which serve to demarcate "The story so far", and to confront the patient with a narrative construction against which to measure the raw material of their experience.

As the therapy proceeds the shaping process becomes less obvious, and is probably most evident in the therapist's rhythms of activity and silence, the balance between verbal interventions, mmmm ... s, grunts, and indrawn breaths. Like an attuned parent, the effective therapist will intuitively sense when the patient needs stimulus and direction to keep the thread of narrative alive, when she needs to be left alone to explore her feelings without intrusion or control. Sometimes, especially when the therapy feels stuck, the therapist may simply describe, or tell the story of what has happened, either in a particular session or sequence of sessions: "You started off today seeming rather sad, and finding it hard to focus, then you began to talk about how difficult you always find Christmas, then you mentioned your friend's aunt who died suddenly." This story may well then provoke a realisation, or moment of insight such as "Oh ... it was Christmas when my grandmother died, I always feel a bit down at this time of year ... maybe that is why ..." This will mark the end of this narrative sequence; the narrative is dispersed, mingled with new experience, until a new narrative sequence emerges.

Implicit in this argument is the view that psychological health (closely linked to secure attachment) depends on a dialectic between story making and story breaking, between the capacity to form narrative, and to disperse it in the light of new experience. In Main's[11] evocative phrase, the securely attached child shows a "fluidity of attentional gaze", and in adult life narrative capacity similarly moves between fluidity and form, between structure and "de-structuring", construction and deconstruction. This capacity ultimately depends on being able to trust both intimacy and aggression[14] – which form the basis of much psychotherapeutic work. Intimacy provides the closeness needed if meaning and experience are to be woven into narrative; trusting one's aggression enables these stories to be broken up and allowed to reform into new patterns. The attachment perspective I have adopted suggests three prototypical pathologies of narrative capacity: clinging to rigid stories; being overwhelmed by unstoried experience; or being unable to find a narrative strong enough to contain traumatic pain.

The role of the therapist

Psychotherapeutic work tests not just the skills of the therapist but also her personal strengths. The therapist's attachment style, and equally her narrative style, will be an all important element in determining the outcome of therapy. Enmeshed therapists tend to impose their own narrative on patients, or get bogged down in interminable stories that have no end, while those with avoidant styles may fail to pick up on vital emotional cues, and jump to unwarranted conclusions. The therapist's task is to be attuned while retaining her balance, a position I have called "non-attachment".[14] Each story is there to be revised in the light of new experience, new facets of memory, new meanings.

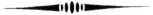

1 Freud S. *The Complete Letters of Sigmund Freud to Wilhelm Fliess: 1887–1905.* Cambridge, MA: Harvard University Press, 1985, p. 160.
2 Wallerstein R. ed. *The Common Ground of Psychoanalysis.* New York: Jason Aronson, 1992.
3 MacIntyre A. *After Virtue.* Notre Dame: University of Notre Dame Press, 1981.
4 Bruner J. *Actual Minds, Possible Worlds.* Cambridge, MA: Harvard University Press, 1986.
5 Phillips J. The Psychoanalytic Narrative. In: Roberts G, Holmes J eds. *Narrative in Psychiatry and Psychotherapy.* Oxford: Oxford University Press, 1998.
6 Spence D. *Narrative Truth and Historical Truth: Meaning and Interpretation in Psychoanalysis.* New York: Norton, 1992.
7 Brockmeier J. Autobiography, narrative and the Freudian conception of life history. *Phil Psychiat Psychol* 1997; 4(3): 201–3.
8 Winnicott D. Mirror-role of mother and family in child development. In: Lomas P. *The Predicament of the Family.* London: Hogarth, 1967.
9 Gergely G, Watson J. The social biofeedback theory of parental affect-mirroring. *Int J Psycho-Anal* 1996; 77: 1181–212.
10 Holmes J. *John Bowlby and Attachment Theory.* London: Routledge, 1993.
11 Main M. Recent studies of attachment: overview with selected implications for clinical work. In: Goldberg S, Muir R, Kerr, J. *Attachment Theory: Social, Developmental and Clinical Perspectives.* Hillsdale, NJ: Analytic Press, 1995.
12 Lacan J. *The Four Fundamental Concepts of Psychoanalysis.* New York: Norton, 1978.
13 Bollas C. *Cracking Up.* London: Routledge, 1995.
14 Holmes J. *Attachment, Intimacy, Autonomy. Using Attachment Theory in Adult Psychotherapy.* New York: Jason Aronson, 1996.

19 The electronic medical record and the "story stuff": a narrativistic model

Stephen Kay and Ian Purves

Introduction

The creation of an "electronic medical record" is claimed to be one of the grand challenges of Medical Informatics.[1] In our scientific community the errant knights who pursue this Holy Grail[2] are committed to eradicating what they see as being the unholy chaos of the paper-based record, replete with untamed narrative. They see, rightly, the many problems caused by poor recording and ineffective retrieval of clinical detail. Amongst the problems they seek to address are the difficulties which arise from clinicians simply misunderstanding illegible script to deeper "integrity faults" related to sins of data omission and commission which result in patients (not only information!) being in the wrong place at the wrong time. What originally was the quest of a few enthusiasts has now become a movement, involving national, European and indeed international standardisation agencies.[3]

This modern day crusade seeks to tame the narrative through the use of the computer by "cleaning up", organising, and formalising both the form and expression of the medical record. The cause is a noble one, but crusades are often dangerous affairs, fixing one problem whilst creating another, and are nearly always guilty of severely disrupting the invaded culture. It is inevitable that the introduction of the computer into the clinical process will, whatever else it does, reorganise the practices of health care. This reorganisation will affect both clinician and patient in many ways, both expected and unforeseen, but with certain implications for the authoring and reading of these soon to be idealised artefacts.[4]

The medical record debate in medical informatics is often

185

fixated on the pros and cons of paper as the preferred medium for the record rather than silicon. In part, what will become of the medical record is to do with what the recording medium will allow, the constraints alluded to in McLuhan's famous dictum, "the medium is the message".[5] There is a sense, however, that if the medical record is considered to be a narrative construct then this narrative must transcend the medium. As Barthes remarks, narratives are "Able to be carried by articulated language, spoken or written, fixed or moving images, gestures, and the ordered mixture of all these substances [...] Moreover, under this almost infinite diversity of forms, narrative is present in every age, in every place, in every society".[6]

Most systems in organisations today, however, are of a hybrid nature, containing a mix of both paper and electronic media with differing proportions of each depending on the requirements of the users. This has led to a spectrum of systems in which the tension between the two types of medium has had to be managed. Undoubtedly the electronic medium in the guise of the computer is becoming more powerful and its science more sophisticated with the result that its representations can more closely approximate what is required. With respect to the electronic medical record's ability to reproduce clinical discourse, some argue that it is already quite close,[7] whilst others argue that it can never be close enough.[8][9] We take the pragmatic view that there are known problems of deficient representation which can be minimised. Specifically, we are attempting to justify why narrative should be re-valued with respect to computer-mediated, patient-serving documentation.

Narrativics and structure

The medical record in our view can be regarded as a particular genre of narrative. Its distinctive nature is derived in part from the clinical situation in which it is constructed, but primarily from the fact that any instance of this genre is a re-construction of a patient's story (or even stories within stories). In addition, the patient's story brings in the clinician(s) so that they, now influential characters in their own right, become part of the plot. Narrative in both its form and expression can capture and convey the richness of this broader story.

It should be emphasised that although our concern is with narrative, we are not opposed to structure. On the contrary we seek to understand the structure of what tends to be denigrated as "free text" in computer-based medical record systems. Rather than regard "free text" as a messy embarrassment to perfect design, or as a last resort to be tolerated when coded forms of formal clinical representation fail, we see it as essential. It is more than "a residual of unrepresentable data and annotation as to the idiosyncratic form in which a given clinician prefers to express himself or herself".[10] More often than not it contains the important "stuff" of the record which we devalue at our peril. In many systems the so-called "free text" is the most useful part of a clinical record. Furthermore there are other sub-genres in medicine, e.g. psychiatry, which thus far have shown little support for the electronic record; their particular focus being too discursive to be easily formalised. "Free text" might usefully be seen as being the difficult bit of a design process that from necessity will always prioritise the simple and achievable first. But as C.S. Lewis reflected with respect to "The Cursings" in the Book of Psalms, "Where we find a difficulty we may always expect a discovery awaits us. Where there is cover we hope for game".[11] We use narratology to examine the difficulties of "free text" with the expectation that we might find what makes a good electronic medical record.

In common with Onega and Landa,[12] we use the term narratology in its broadest etymological sense as a science of narrative, but emphasise the matter of structure that is historically at the root of the subject and is still now regarded as being its core. To them, a narrative is defined as "the representation of a series of events" (p. 5). The narratological framework described in our article "Medical Records and Other Stories"[13] provided us with a comprehensive means of studying the ambivalent nature of narrative, i.e. not only the medical record as a narrative "product" or end result, but also as a narrative "process" which includes the authoring, receiving and the pervasive contextual elements which make up a "good story". With respect to Medical Informatics, the framework permits the consideration of diverse agents initiating and receiving texts, facilitated and filtered by technological media in diverse contexts. In this chapter we focus primarily on the "story product", and the different architectures and technologies which attempt to represent it and make it usable. Narratology as a subject has also come to include such matters but, when talking about the architectures, we prefer to use the more specific term, *Narrativics*, which "develops models accounting for (the structure of) narrative".[14]

As medical informaticians, with computer science and clinical backgrounds, respectively, we are acutely aware of straying into narratological cul de sacs. For example, those concerned with literary criticism may consider our utilitarian viewpoint to be passé and our structuralist emphasis to be flawed and outdated. Structuralism as applied to literary works is less interested in interpreting what literary works mean than in explaining how they mean what they mean; that is, in showing what implicit rules and conventions are operating in a given work. Nethertheless, our defence, in part, is that there is substantial evidence that suggests technology will always lag behind art,[15] and hence there is some value in considering whether structuralist theories can help in our field. Furthermore, narratology can no longer be simply equated to just a structuralist position, as pointed out by Onega, and our work is not just structuralist but has more to do with a deconstruction of clinical narrative. We would cite Culler too, the author of *On Deconstruction*,[16] who argues that deconstruction complements and legitimises structuralist theory rather than demolishes it.[17] What makes the structuralist approach in literature anathema to some critics then, may have considerable value to a scientific culture which pursues only a reductionist approach to problem solving. We have found it useful and believe other scientists will find it credible, even though we regard our present ideas as a beginning rather than an end, and our models as being necessarily provisional at this time.

The model we seek to position is the "narrative medical record". For now, we would claim that it represents a medical record *and* a medical record services both oriented by narrative, situated in a clinical context. As with other models of the medical record it is possible to have many designs and implementations derived from it. Here, though, we consider the architectures, technologies, and associated representations which have contributed to our thinking.

Generations of representing the medical record

Any classification will have a specific purpose and thus select its own view. The explicit purpose of Figure 19.1 is to portray the "technical" development of a medical record from the oral tradition through to logic description, showing that the fabula remains relevant irrespective of how these developments attempt to represent it. By *fabula* we mean the basic story material, "the set of

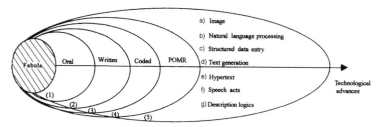

Figure 19.1   The relevance of fabula to five generations of the medical record (POMR = problem oriented medical record)

narrated situations and events in their chronological sequence",[19] or simply the "story stuff".[20] (We prefer this vague expression as it does not seem to prejudge whether fabula is the truly "raw material" of the story or an abstract concept or product emerging from tensions within the narrative.)

Our time-line shows successive generations of the medical record culminating in the fifth, today's "new wave". Each new generation of the record implies some criticism of its predecessor and is supported in its critique by new advances in technology. In situated health care, many of these "generations" will coexist and some will not yet have been heard of in the majority of settings. None is universally accepted either in terms of usage (which to an extent is dependent upon culture, organisation, and resource) or in terms of acknowledged support (which to an extent is dependent on politics, ideology, and presentation). The more recent developments like the structured data entry and description logics which are introduced later, for example, are approaches that are only now beginning to emerge from the research laboratories and become commercially available.

Technologies and the narrative in the medical record

Although some of these new areas in the fifth generation are more recent than others, it is not yet clear whether the developments are complete or are still active in a developmental process, nor is it clear quite what their relationship to each other is. These recent developments arise in part from a critique of their peer technologies and in part from an understanding of new requirements related to the medical record. To speak of predecessors and successors in these areas is clearly premature. It is perhaps important to remember that 1948 was the birth of the first stored program computer in Manchester[21] and that in contrast to, say, the earliest oral tradition, this latest generation of the medical record is still very immature. It is also likely that the future medical record will be a manifestation of a combination of such approaches, and for these reasons we group them along the timeline in the same "wave". The different developments in Figure 19.1 are briefly considered next with a view to establishing the importance of the narrative medical record in relation to these technologies. The remaining part of this chapter is structured around the diverse types of representation shown in Figure 19.1.

1. *The oral record* (not dictation) is stored in the human memory and transmitted by speech. The oral record is localised, dying with the original individual unless passed on beforehand. The record is only kept alive by telling and re-telling the patient's story.

2. *The written record*, however, can persist beyond the limitations of the originator and the originating context. Whether oral or written, both forms give the opportunity of improvement through narrative analysis.[22] For example, Coulthard[23] analysed and evaluated a pamphlet of the British Diabetic Association, entitled *Holidays and Travel for Diabetics*, in response to a plea from a nurse who claimed that "our patients can't understand this". Although there are various attempts to standardise the medical record, both oral and written records might best be characterised at this time as being *ad hoc* representations, independent of common standards of form and layout. Until the computer appeared, similarities between records were apparently explained by chance and perhaps by reference to an institutional or professions' preferred "house style".

3. Conventional medical informatics became interested in the development of the *coded record* once the computer became the medium by which such records were represented and expressed. Paper based, handwritten records were perceived as being problematic both for individual patient care and for other secondary purposes which were coming to the fore (e.g. resource management). Ironically, there is a danger that "paper" may disappear before we discover its successes. The first "replacements", i.e. initial computer based records, were severely constrained by the technology that spawned them. For reasons of efficiency (e.g. expensive storage and processing

constraints; time and effort for user interaction), as well as clinical efficacy, various clinical coding systems were developed. In the UK, perhaps the earliest, most comprehensive set of codes were developed in General Practice by Perry.[24] It was when such coding systems were found to be insufficient for the clinician's needs, the system designers offered "free text" to permit a richer expression of the clinical data. Despite the claimed potential advantages of the computer based approach, and some implicit structuring given by the underlying coding system, these records were often retrograde compared to the paper version. Not only did they consist of *ad hoc*, unstructured recordings dependent upon the situation, but the system and its design imposed its own limited view upon the discourse. Until then, there had been no successful attempt to consider the broader picture, and to organise the content of the medical record to reflect how clinicians perform their day to day routine work.

4. A watershed for Medical Informatics was the innovation of a framework or model by Laurence Weed.[25] His *Problem Oriented Medical Record (POMR)* was an attempt to tame the wild excesses of narrative, to provide a medical record which was designed for the computer which would become "the principal reference tool ... by coupling medical knowledge to medical action with a precision never before considered possible".[26] In response, many believed that a fully electronic patient record was imminent even though the technology at that time only provided primitive support for the simplest of tasks and severely limited interaction between machine and user. Many systems including Weed's own, PROMIS, however, were built around the elusive idea of "the problem". Whilst acknowledging the major contribution made by Weed, some began to question the practicality of his model.[27] To them, the POMR was too prescriptive, requiring the clinician to modify his or her "natural" behaviour, and was less suited to non-hospital domains. General Practice in particular posed significant difficulties for the implementation where "problems" emerged messily over extended periods of time rather than being presented fully formed. POMR is too neat, and an impressive example of how structures can "clean up" after the event. Consider the aptly named SOAP, where the patient's contribution is *subjective* and the clinicians' *objective*! Similar glosses and "smooth flows" can be found in other non-clinical, office

procedures as highlighted by Suchman,[28] "Standard procedures are formulated in the interest of what things should come to, and not necessarily how they should arrive there". However, the POMR is still perhaps the only widely recognised conceptual framework specifically designed for clinical purposes even in the present "new wave", and is one which might be considered to transcend the various media by articulating the "problem" as the focus of clinical attention.

5. The following are fifth generation of medical record representations:

(a) *Image* is the first of the representations considered in the new generation of the electronic medical record. The interest in image is more than just the fact that in clinical settings the film is usually accompanied by a text report. It is a pervasive technology which is included in monitoring applications, such as people watching (e.g. in wards and in homes), as well as the more common management of paper documents. Indeed, the scanning of documents gives substance to the cliché, "Every picture tells a story". Chatman has gone further and shown in his book entitled *Story and Discourse: Narrative Structure in Fiction and Film*[19] that the media differences do not diminish the relevance of narratology. This is particularly important, as imaging technology is perhaps the most accepted innovation to date in the fifth generation as it includes radiology in its realm of influence as well as document scanning. Simulation, visualisation and, further on, virtual reality research are also allied to this area, and the latter has already been found to be explicated by reference to the visual arts.[29] These technologies are now being researched in theory as well as being applied to the health care domain in practice.

(b) *Natural Language Processing (NLP)* is an approach in the new generation that returns the attention back to more traditional forms of narrative. It researches the means by which natural language can be analysed and captured by computer. Its increasing sophistication owes much to the development of the technology, be it focused upon speech or text,[30 31] and it is extremely important for what we are calling the narrative medical record. Natural language processing technology was first applied to the clinical domain as a reactive response to the poor uptake of the computer by clinicians for direct entry of their notes by a keyboard. Thus, natural language processing and analysis of medical language has usually been motivated by the consideration of the presence of the ubiquitous paper based record. Given this paper record, what do we do with it?

(c) By contrast, the more recent *Structured Data Entry*[32] is intended to facilitate direct entry of clinical data by the clinician, often by reducing the dependency upon keyboard skills. An example from the *Clinergy GP* system is given in Figure 19.2. Structured data entry is built around the idea of descriptions and it is sufficiently flexible so as not to prescribe how data is entered into the system by the clinician. This to some extent overcomes some of the difficulties associated with POMR. This approach is made possible by new innovations such as the graphical user interface with point and click metaphors, powerful hardware, and sophisticated software languages. The result is that the medical record is entered into the system by a series of structured forms. Free text may still be present in these

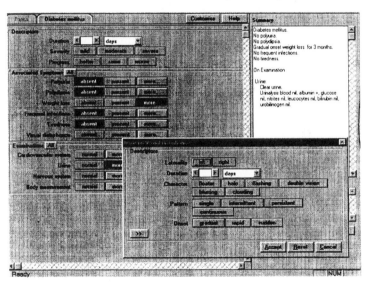

Figure 19.2   The form, "Visual disturbance", is shown when the clinician points to the 'more ...' button. Entering detail in the form will result in that button being highlighted. The details selected will appear as structured text within the record Summary (illustrated by the "Weight loss" detail shown in the top, right corner of the figure).

systems and can complement the form based input, yet more of the clinical detail is expected to be (and can be) expressed by formal means in the structured data entry system than in the earlier systems. Interestingly, usability[33] was originally the main motivation for structured data entry, the descriptive approach giving the user (author/reader) more freedom to express and see detail as required. Further enhancements led to modelling the medical record, so that not only were the recorded statements clinically sensible but the forms themselves contained only that which was clinically relevant for the clinician's specific purpose. This predictive form[34] was still based upon the descriptive approach but only implicitly considered process and the wider context. Although structured data entry is recognised as being superior to many of the current data entry approaches, there are subtle dangers if it becomes the only way of capturing data. Structured data entry alone, through making some data entry tasks easier than others (e.g. describing anatomical site as opposed to psycho-social matters), will re-enforce what McWhinney calls the dualistic division between body and mind.[35] As these technologies become part of the changing consultation it is important that they should add value for the patient as well as the clinician.[36 37]

(d) *Text Generation*, or more generally Natural Language Generation (NLG), is an approach which is concerned with the output of text rather than with data entry. As such, it adds value more to the audience of the medical record than to the author. Given that part of the record may have to be shown or told to a non-implied reader, perhaps for litigation or for education purposes, NLG can develop customised pieces of text. These texts might be suitable for, say, patient advice[38] or for informing clinicians from other specialties in the form of referral or discharge letters. As an example of its application to legal use, patients in the UK have a right of access to an explained version of their medical record. In these instances what is generated may only be a partial record or an explanation of part of it. In cases where the underlying representation of the record is unsuitable for direct presentation,[39 40] NLG can make what is presented to the reader much more readable. It can also be seen as part of a broader narratological framework.[41] Weed himself, back in 1973, regarded it as self evident that patients should have a personal copy of the medical record for purposes of feedback and quality control

> The providers should be working for the day when [the patient] could see his complete list of problems, could see clearly what our plans were for each problem and be able to see the carefully constructed Progress Notes for each problem. He, too, then could discern the patterns of our thoughts – our priorities – and the results, good and bad, of what we do.[42]

We are still working for that day and NLG it is argued may have an important part to play in speeding its arrival. A recent review by Cawsey et al [43] considers the different types of NLG and the motivation for continuing research in this area. Natural language generation shares some of the characteristics and the potential found in natural language processing, referred to earlier. Despite this, however, it is still rarely found within current health care settings.

(e) *Hypertext* applications, by contrast, are becoming increasingly common, both in local manifestations and in global ones such as are afforded by the internet and the World Wide Web. Flexibility, particularly with respect to navigable access, has made it an obvious approach for the medical record, or at least for specific aspects of the medical record. McLellan points out that narratives of physical illness are being constructed by patients and that authoring by multiple narrators is becoming a hallmark of this new medium.[44] Soetikno et al [45] describe how the Web is used for quality-of-life research providing autobiographical patient accounts of ulcerative colitis. It is the technology and its "push", however, which has made hypertext approaches so popular and ubiquitous. The use of hypertext in the medical record suffers from a lack of theoretical underpinning and applications vary tremendously with respect to quality. Here too narrative science,[46] and particularly those elements within it related to rhetoric,[47] are poised to play an important part in future developments, although there is then a need to further "link" this work to the clinical domain. Box 19.1 shows an early example of how some of the approaches in the fifth generation of medical records rely on a combination of tools rather than an exclusive approach. PIGLET (Personalised Intelligent Generator of

Little Explanatory Texts) is an example of an architecture which encompasses both simple NLG and hypertext approaches using information within the patient record to customise the explanation. Words in **bold** type in Box 19.1 (from Binsted *et al.*[48]) can be touched or clicked to disclose more information. Text within the angled brackets has been added.

(f) Hypertexts considered as multi-authored, collaborative works are also our re-entry here into the field of communication and the study of language. In much the same way as we seek to apply narrativics to medical records, others have sought to find ways of using and generating new frameworks through "language as action" approaches. *Speech Acts* and theories from Austin[49] and Searle[50] are attempts to formalise the informal and are concerned with the logic behind linguistic behaviour. In this light, some see

---

Box 19.1: Language Generation and HyperText in one application.

< Problems recorded in Mark Smith's record >
Type one diabetes mellitus Diagnosed: 1965.
Angina pectoris Diagnosed: 1975.
Background diabetic retinopathy Diagnosed: 1988.
Nephrotic syndrome Diagnosed: 1988.
Hyperlipidaemia Diagnosed: 1992.

< If Mark opts to see an explanation of Hyperlipidaemia then the following text of generalised and personalised information is displayed:
>
HYPERLIPIDAEMIA
"Hyperlipidaemia" is the term for having a high level of lipids (fats), particularly cholesterol, in the blood. According to your **record**, you have this problem. Possible causes include *family history*, **diabetes mellitus** and **high alcohol intake**. Some common treatments include a special diet and **a lipid-lowering drug**. It increases the risk of **atherosclerosis** and **coronary artery disease**. Your cholesterol level was last measured at 3.8 mmol/L (15 July 1994). You have a lipid-lowering drug in your record: **bezafibrate**.

< If Mark now wished to find out more about the drug bezafibrate then a click on the last word would link him to a screen which would describe the nature of the drug and provide guide-lines for how Mark should use it. >

---

clinical recording as primarily a problem of effective co-ordination rather than as a requirement for the definitive, comprehensive medical record architecture. Certainly the need to share records across professional boundaries for clinical purposes is apparent in the call for more team working involving clinicians and the patient. Consequently, Groupware, Workflow and Co-ordination systems are now perceived as being important for clinical settings.[51] The inclusion of speech acts, however, is to emphasise the very close relationship between narrative and language approaches generally. In some senses we are returning to the oral and written record; at least we now have the potential to analyse clinical discourse by means of conversation analysis and discourse analysis through ethnographic and technical means, and to consider philosophies of communication (e.g. Habermas) as possible pointers to the future.[52] This area also highlights the tensions between schools of thought that range from socio-political issues surrounding decisions and choice[53] to Discursive Psychology[54] that challenges the traditional perception of the "communication model" and "representation".

(g) The last approach in this analysis is that of Description Logics. In the clinical arena, there is a clear link from the structured data entry (referred to above), which is based upon descriptions, to the terminological considerations addressed in description logic.[55] GRAIL,[56] is the description logic driving the type of dialogue given in Figure 19.2 and is responsible for constraining the details which appear on the form and thus determines what can be entered by a clinician; a model represents what is 'clinically sensible' and the appropriate data entry form is generated accordingly. Like Austin's and Searle's work when applied to health care it seeks to bring a logic to the task of creating useful and usable formalisms. Description logic is mathematical and consequently its output is more rigorous as well as more specialised. It will be active behind the scenes of the medical record rather than frontstage. For example, GRAIL is used to structure the knowledge base in more recent versions of PIGLET for generating natural language. Narrative, at least in literary theory, is held to be a higher concept than description.[57] Description, however, has been proven to work as a foundation to electronic medical records;[58–60] now it is the turn of narrative to see whether or not it can make a further contribution to Medical Informatics theory.

The problem and the story

Often it is claimed that "technology for health care is no longer a problem, rather it is merely a management problem that has to be solved". Whilst not wishing to play down organisational issues, the review of the above technologies for the medical record has shown that we are at the start rather than at the end of the technological road. We are still a long way off from regaining the richness of what we have (had) in paper whilst being able to benefit or add value from the new technologies.

The narratological framework which we developed has permitted us to (re-)discover the role that narrative plays in the medical record irrespective of the medium used to represent it. As with the other developments, the narrative medical record will require a mixture of existing and new forms of technology to function effectively. This model however permits the investigation of semantics external to the document itself, permits consideration of the agents and processes which surround it, and situates the communicative context. Furthermore, it has an array of analytical tools to consider both the internal and external properties based upon a wealth of mature literary theories. The narrative medical record has the potential to remove the hard distinction between psychosomatic diseases and others by treating the discursive elements and the more directly measurable elements with equal respect. It is perhaps a new development[61], a "healing art"[62] that facilitates a "new language which speaks of the mind-body, not the mind *and* the body".[35] To propose fabula (i.e. the story stuff) to be fundamentally intrinsic to medicine we are following the path marked out by Weed in relation to "Problem". However, whereas the "tame" problem has arguably failed in clinical practice, at least in those parts which require a more discursive approach, the available riches that we can draw upon within narratology means that the "wild" narrative or even the *freed* text might come to succeed.

Acknowledgment

The forms which are shown in Figure 19.2 are courtesy of Semantic Technologies Limited who develop and market the *Clinergy GP* system.

1 Sittig DF. Grand Challenges in Medical Informatics. *J Am Med Inform Assoc* 1994; **1**: 412–13.

2 Dick RS, Gabler J. Still Searching for the Holy Grail. *Health Management Technol* 1995: 30–80.

3 McDonald CJ. ANSI's Health Informatics Planning Panel – The purpose and progress. In: De Moor GJE, McDonald CJ, Noothoven van Goor J eds. *Progress in Standardisation in Health Care Informatics*. Amsterdam: IOS Press, 1993, pp. 14–19.

4 Berg M. Practices of reading and writing: the constitutive role of the patient record in medical work. *Soc Health Illness* 1996; **18**(4): 499–524.

5 McLuhan M, Powers BR. *The Global Village: The Transformation in World Life and Media in the 21st Century*. Oxford: Oxford University Press, 1989.

6 Barthes R. Introduction to the Structural Analysis of Narratives. In: Onega S, Landa JAG. *Narratology*. New York: Longman, 1996, p. 46.

7 Kluge EHW. Advanced patient records: some ethical and legal considerations touching medical informatics space. *Meth Inform Med* 1993; **32**: 95–103.

8 Button G, Coulter J, Lee JRE, Sharrock W. *Computers, Minds and Conduct*. Cambridge: Polity Press, 1995.

9 Grémy F, Leplège A, Hève D. The computerized medical record is not the patient analog. A four partners scenario in clinical encounters. *Meth Inform Med* 1993; **32**: 339–40.

10 Rector AL. Marking up is not enough. *Meth Inform Med* 1993; **32**: 272.

11 Lewis CS. *Reflections on the Psalms*. London: Fontana Books, 1972. p. 29.

12 Onega S, Landa JAG. *Narratology*. New York: Longman, 1996.

13 Kay S, Purves IN. Medical Records and Other Stories: a narratological framework. *Meth Inform Med*. 1996; **35**: 72–88.

14 Prince G. *Dictionary of Narratology*. Aldershot: Scolar Press, 1993, p. 64.

15 Schlain L. *Art and Physics: Parallel visions in space, time and light*. New York: William Morrow and Company, 1991.

16 Culler J. *On Deconstruction. Theory and Criticism after Structuralism*. London: Routledge & Kegan Paul, 1982.

17 Culler J. *Saussure*. London: Fontana Press. 1985.

18 Prince G. *Dictionary of Narratology*. Aldershot: Scolar Press, 1993.

19 Chatman S. *Story and Discourse: Narrative Structure in Fiction and Film*. Cornell University Press, 1978. p. 19.

20 COMPUTER 50, http://www/computer50.org .

21 Riessman CK. *Narrative Analysis*. Newbury Park, CA: Sage Publications, 1993.

22 Coulthard M. On analysing and evaluating written text. In: Coulthard M *Advances in written text analysis*. London: Routledge, 1994.

23 Perry J. Records for Clinical Care and Epidemiology. In: Symposium on Automated records in primary care. Oxford Community Health Project, 1980, Y1–Y10.

24 Weed LL. *Medical Records, Medical Education and Patient Care*. Cleveland: The Press of Case Western Reserve University, 1971.

25 Weed LL. Quality Control. In: Walker HK, Hurst JW, Woody MF eds. *Applying the problem-oriented system*. New York: MEDCOM Press, 1973, p. 8.

26 Rector AL, Kay S. Descriptive Models for Medical Records and Data Interchange. In: Barber B, Cao D, Qin D, Wagner G eds *MEDINFO 89*. Amsterdam: North Holland, 1989, 230–4.

27 Suchman LA. Office Procedure as Practical Action: Models of Work and System Design. *ACM Trans Office Inform Systems*, 1983; **1**(4): 320–8.

28 Chatman S. *Story and Discourse: Narrative structure in fiction and film*. Ithaca, NY: Cornell University Press, 1993.

29 Laurel B. *Computers as Theatre*. Reading, MA: Addison-Wesley, 1993.

30 Sager N, Friedman C, Lyman MS. *Medical Language Processing: Computer*

management of narrative data. Reading, MA: Addison-Wesley, 1987; p. 24.

31 Bateman J, Teich E. *Selective information presentation in an integrated publication system: an application of genre-driven text generation.* 1994.

32 Howkins TJ, Kay S, Rector AL, Goble CA, Horan B, Nowlan WA , Wilson A. An Overview of the PEN & PAD Project. In: O'Moore R, Bengtsson S, Bryant JR, Bryden JS eds, *Medical Notes in Medical Informatics No.40 MIE 90,* Berlin: Springer-Verlag, 1990; 73–8.

33 Horan B *et al.* Supporting a humanly impossible task: The clinical human-computer environment. In: *Interact 90.* Amsterdam: Elsevier, 1990; 247–52.

34 Rector AL, Nowlan WA. Predictive Data Entry. In: *AIME-91.* Berlin: Springer-Verlag, 1991.

35 McWhinney IR. The Importance of being different. *Brit J Gen Pract* 1996; **46**: 433–6.

36 Kay S, Horan B, Goble CA, Howkins TJ, Rector AL, Nowlan A, Wilson A. A Consulting Room System with Added Value. In: O'Moore R, Bengtsson S, Bryant JR, Bryden JS eds, *Medical Notes in Medical Informatics No.40 MIE 90,* Berlin: Springer-Verlag, 1990; pp. 73–8.

37 Purves IN. The Changing Consultation. In: van Zwanenberg T, Harrison J eds. *GP Tomorrow.* Oxford: Radcliffe Medical Press, 1998, pp. 31–47.

38 Carenini G, Mittal VO, Moore JD. Generating patient-specific interactive natural language explanations. In: Cawsey A ed., *AI Patient Education.* Glasgow: GIST Technical Report: G95.3, 1995; 39–43.

39 Bullock JC. Text generation from semantic network based medical records. MSc Thesis, University of Manchester, Department of Computer Science, 1994.

40 Bullock JC, Solomon D. Generating Narratives from Medical Records. In: Cawsey A ed., *AI in Patient Education.* Glasgow: GIST Technical Report: G95.3, 1995; 23–6.

41 Kay S, Bullock JC. Generation of clinical narrative: PEN&PAD: Reporter and Story. In: Richards B ed. *Proceedings of Healthcare Computing, Harrogate,* 1996; 513–20.

42 Weed LL. Quality Control. In: Walker HK, Hurst JW, Woody MF eds. *Applying the problem-oriented system.* New York: MEDCOM Press, 1973; p. 5.

43 Cawsey AJ, Webber BL, Jones RB. Natural Language Generation in Health Care. *J Am Med Inform Assoc* 1997; **4**: 473–82.

44 McLellan MF. Literature and medicine: narratives of physical illness. *Lancet* 1997; **349**: 1618–20.

45 Soetikno RM, Mrad R, Pao V, Lenert LA. Quality-of-life Research on the Internet: Feasibility and Potential Biases in Patients with Ulcerative Colitis. *J Am Med Inform Assoc* 1997; **4**: 426–35.

46 Aarseth EJ. Nonlinearity and Literary Theory. In: Landow GP ed. *Hyper/Text/Theory.* Baltimore: John Hopkins University Press, 1994; pp. 51–86.

47 Landow GP. What is a critic to do?: Critical theory in the age of Hypertext. In: Landow GP ed. *Hypertext theory.* Baltimore: John Hopkins University Press, 1994, 1–50.

48 Binsted K, Cawsey A, Jones R. Generating Personalised Patient Information Using the Medical Record, AI in Patient Education (AIPE) August 1995. *GIST Technical Report: G95.3.*

49 Austin J. *How to do things with words.* Oxford: Oxford University Press, 1962.

50 Searle J. *Speech Acts.* Cambridge: Cambridge University Press, 1969.

51 Purves IN. Decision support at the primary/secondary care interface. In: Pritchard P ed. *Decision support in primary and secondary care.* London: NHS Executive R&D, 1987, pp. 33–41.

52 Schoop M. Habermas and Searle in Hospital: a description Language for Cooperative Documentation systems in Healthcare. In: Dignum F, Dietz J eds. *Communication Modelling – The Language/Action Perspective.* Report 97-09, Eindhoven: Eindhoven University of Technology, 1997, pp. 117–32.

53 Suchman L. Do categories have Politics?: The language/action perspective reconsidered. *Computer Supported Cooperative Work (CSCW)*, 1994; **2**(3): 177–90.
54 Edwards D. *Discourse and Cognition*. London: Sage Publications, 1997.
55 Rogers JE, Rector AL. Terminological Systems: Bridging the Generation Gap. In: Masys DR ed. *Proceedings 1997 AMIA Fall Symposium*. Philadelphia: Hanley & Belfus, 1997, pp. 610–14.
56 Rector AL, Nowlan WA, Glowinski A. Goals for concept representation in the GALEN Project. In: Safran C ed. *Proceedings of the Seventeenth Annual Symposium on Computer Applications in Medical Care*, Washington, DC. New York: McGraw-Hill, 1994; pp. 414–18.
57 Prince G. *Narrative. Dictionary of Narratology*. Aldershot: Scolar Press, 1987, 57–8.
58 Rector AL, Nowlan WA, Kay S. Unifying Medical Information using an Architecture Based on Descriptions. In: Miller RA ed. *Proceedings of the Symposium on Computer Applications in Medical Care, SCAMC 90, Washington*, 1990, pp. 190–4.
59 Rector AL, Nowlan WA, Kay S. Foundations for an Electronic Medical Record. *Meth Inform Med* 1991; **30**: 179–86.
60 Rector AL, Nowlan WA, Kay S, Goble CA, Howkins TJ. A framework for modelling the electronic medical record. *Meth Inform Med* 1992; **32**(2): 109–19.
61 Grémy F, Lelaidier, Hève D. Is there anything new about the so-called "medical" record? *Meth Inform Med* 1996; **35**: 93–7.
62 Smith BH, Taylor RJ. Medicine – a healing or a dying art? *Brit J Gen Pract* 1996; **46**: 249–51.

20 Anecdote in clinical practice

Jane Macnaughton

Introduction

The "deceptive power" of the anecdote lies in the fact that single startling cases (the stuff of anecdote) stick in the mind.[1] Whereas textbook accounts of illness tend to focus upon typical presentations, anecdotes tell us what is not typical and provide us with decidedly skewed views of medicine.[2] Nevertheless, doctors cannot resist telling such stories: the "I remember a patient once..." scenario[3] pervades medical meetings and teaching rounds and serves important and useful functions.

What are anecdotes?

The word "anecdote" is used in two senses. The first can be found in the sentence, "I would like to tell you a story (i.e. an anecdote) about ...", and the second in "That's purely anecdotal!" The first sense indicates the primary meaning of the word; the speaker is about to tell a short story illustrating a point in a more dramatic way than merely stating it. The second sense is more dismissive. For example, a doctor may respond to a story about the efficacy of some new treatment with "That's purely anecdotal". The implication is, "That's just a story, we need to look for the *real* evidence elsewhere".

Two examples illustrate the distinguishing features of anecdotes. The first is stand-up comedians, who depend heavily on anecdote for their material. Their stories are short, often fictional ("reality embellished"), culminating in a dramatic punchline which produces a laugh. Anecdote used for humour depends on a shared culture and identity with particular groups, as illustrated by the wedding speech where the audience is usually composed of family and close friends who share a common knowledge about the couple.

Anecdotes are also frequently found in the obituary pages of the newspapers. Here is an extract from an obituary of an English painter who died recently:

> ... though he had his moments of ready conviviality he never really belonged to the art world. Possibly his personal background had something to do with this. He was born into a working class family in Lancashire ... . It is recorded that when his father asked him what he thought he wanted to do for a living, and he answered that he wanted to be a painter, his father was very happy, assuming that what he wanted to paint was houses.[4]

The obituary differs from biography in that it must give a brief account of the person's life, with some (usually flattering) reference to their character. Often included in obituaries as amusing and memorable stories about the person's life anecdotes also serve, as here, to illustrate or account for a trait of character. Here the painter's humble origins are told, the anecdote about his father's mistake serving to illustrate that his origins and upbringing were sufficiently prosaic to make him less inclined to join in with the parties and glamour of the art world.

From these examples of the non-medical use of anecdotes we can see that several features characterise this form of narrative:

1. Anecdotes are short stories with a single theme or point to make. As such, unlike other sorts of narrative such as novels and biography, they cannot involve plot or character development.
2. They may be fictional, non-fictional, or "reality embellished" to add interest or emphasis.
3. Anecdotes often have a dramatic or amusing content illustrative of something moral or educational, or of an amusing aspect of an individual's character.
4. The aim of telling an anecdote is usually to enable the audience to remember or understand the general point being made.
5. This understanding is facilitated if the anecdote is told in vernacular terms and in a context where the audience shares a common background or culture.

Given these defining features, not all of which may be present in every anecdote, it is not surprising that "anecdotal evidence" is accorded limited credibility in scientific circles. Such evidence is often rightly dismissed as a short, dramatic and memorable story told for effect and liable to be embellished! Nevertheless, these very features of the anecdote constitute its potential strengths as well as its widely acknowledged limitations.

Experiential learning: knowledge as accumulated anecdote

A newly qualified doctor has a great deal of factual knowledge but is often a poor decision maker. Practical professional knowledge (what to *do* about particular cases) is a complex phenomenon that is difficult to deconstruct into a set of component competencies.[5] It has been demonstrated that doctors learn primarily through the accumulation of stories about individual patients, sometimes referred to as "illness scripts".[6] This term describes knowledge built up through clinical experience of patients with differing diseases and treatment regimens.

It is thought that, on a mostly subconscious level, doctors compare the patient in front of them with the remembered "illness script" of a previous patient with a similar illness. Any differences between the two stories can lead the doctor to do further investigations or seek additional evidence or advice on the case.[7] Because doctors are likely to remember the more atypical patient story, and those with unusual or striking problems, and because of the haphazard nature of personal experience, learning by anecdote clearly needs to be supplemented by other, more systematic, sources of evidence. Nevertheless, the centrality of the anecdote as a means to what physicians know[8] should be recognised as a reality by those who seek to educate the profession.

Anecdote based medicine: storytelling between doctors

Whenever doctors get together, however formally or informally, anecdotes are recounted. One good reason for this is that everyone enjoys such stories. They enliven dull conference proceedings and serious medical meetings, and are so much a part of communication between doctors that one literary critic has commented that their ubiquity must surely be a manifestation of medical instinct at work. Katherine Montgomery Hunter notes that:

the smaller and more regular the group and the more its members are engaged in the same clinical activities, the more anecdotes will be told.[9]

The kind of setting described here is most likely to be a ward round, hospital unit or a general practice case conference. In formal settings such as at conferences, hospital meetings and in journals these stories have an illustrative function. At a conference presentation, alongside the scientific data on a new therapy for example, a case may be cited as an example of how well the therapy worked. The cited case is usually one in which the therapy worked particularly well, or alternatively, a case in which the therapy was a complete failure.

As we have seen, anecdotes do not recount the commonplace but serve to illustrate the best and the worst of the therapy in addition to the scientific evidence. In this setting, therefore, anecdotes have a role in drawing our attention to the promise and pitfalls of new treatments. And in discussion which follows a conference, the audience will often advance anecdotes to provide counter-examples to what has been presented: "Your patient may have responded in that way but I tried that in a patient of mine once and she ... nearly died." Because anecdotes by their nature are memorable, one told by a speaker may stimulate the memory of another in the audience producing a discussion on the usefulness of a therapy under different circumstances in another patient.

These examples point to the value of anecdotes in continuing medical education as they provide real examples and counter-examples on which practising doctors hone and test their medical knowledge. Anecdote swapping also enables doctors to test their clinical judgment against that of their peers. But anecdotes are also frequently used in undergraduate medical education where clinical teaching goes on around the bed of a patient with a particular illness and clinical signs. Frequently the clinician who is doing the teaching will make reference by anecdote to other similar cases for comparison. Besides this, the teacher will also put forward hypothetical situations such as, "What if this patient *had* had a heart attack? How would this change your management?" These scenarios we might regard as anecdotes about hypothetical cases serving to extend the educational value of a single case.[10]

Anecdotes are often told to students about the great medical figures of the past to illustrate the importance of some very basic medical truth. One such example is a story told of Sir James

Mackenzie, a general practitioner and pioneer in the field of cardiology in the early part of this century:

> Mackenzie was making a weekend visit to his university city of Edinburgh. A surgeon invited him to give his opinion on the circulatory condition of a woman in a ward at the Infirmary, awaiting cholecystectomy. She was found to have anomalous heart sounds. This had aroused doubt in the surgeon's mind about the wisdom of operating. The news of Mackenzie's visit had spread and a crowd of staff and students gathered in the ward. He talked to her about her home. It was on the top floor of a house in the Lawn Market. Did she shop for her family of six? Of course, who else? And carry it up the stairs? Indeed, yes. And how many times a day did she climb those stairs? Countless times. And did she find them trying? Why should she? Mackenzie turned to the surgeon and told him to operate with confidence so far as the function of the heart was concerned.[11]

As well as having a role in education, anecdotes are of undoubted help in the induction of doctors into the etiquette of the profession.[12] Hospital residents, for instance, will seek advice from their predecessor on the preferred procedures in a new ward. Advice is frequently given in the form of a professionalising anecdote of the warning type: "make sure you do this if this ..." or "don't do that because ...", but anecdotes can also provide a much needed support function. Medicine is not very good as a profession at providing formal support for practitioners when they have made mistakes or misjudgments. Case conferences and ward or practice meetings may provide this help in the form of a supportive anecdote. A junior partner in our practice was upset at having missed a case of tuberculosis in a young slim patient with a cough. The senior partner responded: "It's easily done. I did the same thing with a woman whom I thought was anorexic and then she suddenly coughed up blood and had to be rushed into hospital!" "We've all done it" is an expression frequently heard when doctors admit their mistakes to their colleagues and there frequently follows an account of another's mistake with the reassurance that "it can happen to us all". These supportive accounts do not just amount to crying on one another's shoulders, they usually lead to a shared learning experience.

Anecdotes in journals: case reports as evidence

Though not a substitute for systematic scientific research, anecdotes can be the "lateral thinking" which helps to point research in new directions. Single case reports in medical journals often describe puzzling cases which do not quite fit the prevailing scientific knowledge. Such anomalies can serve to stimulate further research and discovery in medicine, particularly when doctors working in the same field find that they are picking up similar anomalies and a series of cases starts to emerge. The written anecdote in the form of a single case report or an account appearing under "A memorable patient" section of the *British Medical Journal* can serve the important role of stimulating investigation.

One famous example cited by Hunter was the outbreak of phocomelia (limb shortening defects) subsequently found to be associated with the drug thalidomide used for morning sickness in pregnancy.[13] A more recent example is concern over the possible dangers of silicone breast implants. The Yellow Card scheme for reporting adverse drug reactions to the UK Committee on Safety of Medicines[14] is a formal mechanism for collecting and aggregating doctors' anecdotal reports about single patients who are thought to have suffered significant side effects or adverse reactions from medication.

Anecdotes and randomised controlled trials can come together in the case of the so-called "N of 1" study, an internally randomised study in an individual patient.[15] Such trials may be used to answer a clinical dilemma concerning a particular patient. Two different treatments (most commonly, an active drug and a placebo) are systematically varied and the response to each one documented. The aim of such a study is to prove or disprove the effectiveness of each treatment *in this particular patient*. The reporting of such a "trial" in turn becomes an anecdote as it fulfils all the necessary features described above.[16]

Anecdote in the consultation

Patients use anecdote as their chief medium for explaining why they have come to consult. In the general practice setting, patients' accounts of their problems are generally undifferentiated and unmedicalised because they have not yet had their story reinterpreted by a doctor. For instance, angina is not yet "A tight pain in my chest which I get with exertion", it is still described in this way:

> The reason I am here, doctor, is that last week I was walking to the shops with my wife and we came back with a lot of

> shopping and had to climb up the hill to the house because the bus broke down. As we reached the top of the hill I suddenly got this pain in my chest which made me stop and gasp for breath.

Anecdotes are also used by patients to illustrate how particular symptoms are affecting their lives. This is a recent exchange I had with a patient who is particularly keen on the game of bowls:

> RJM: How are the knees just now? Are the new painkillers working better?
> MM: Oh no, it's just as bad doctor, and with me Lady President of the bowling green this season too.
> RJM: How are you getting on with the bowling?
> MM: Oh, I'm not able to play just now. The last time I had a match I tried to deliver a bowl and I couldn't get up again! Some of the men had to lift me up off the green. It gave everyone a good laugh but I haven't been able to play since.

This kind of patient anecdote is important because it reflects that individual's experience of the problem and gives the doctor a clear idea of how function is affected. For MM, mild osteoarthritis of the knees was having a major impact on her lifestyle and merited physiotherapy and an orthopaedic surgeon's opinion. For another elderly woman whose lifestyle was not so active the condition might not have prompted any action. The anecdote reminds us that what the patient is interested in is their ability to function, not the severity or otherwise of the pathology.

Patients' illustrative anecdotes can also be revealing of their understanding or misunderstanding of a suspected illness. A patient who had a urostomy scar that had developed a herniation told me:

> But my Uncle James had his hernias operated on down here [indicating her groin area]. I thought it was only men that had hernias. Mind you my sister has one up here inside [indicating the epigastric area] and she has problems eating with it.

This series of anecdotes reveals the patient's (reasonable) confusion over the idea of a hernia and how it can exist in several different places. Paying attention to patient anecdote allows doctors the chance to clarify areas of misunderstanding and become aware of how patients perceive their illness and their own ability to do something about it.

Anecdotes about other patients may be told to patients by doctors as reassurance or as an example of how long symptoms are likely to last. Anecdotes in this context may have limited success as patients may not be interested in someone else's experience of the same illness, especially if it is perceived as being different from their own.

Anecdote in folk models of illness

It is not just in the conference hall or the doctor's surgery where anecdotes are used to communicate on medical matters. Patients share their own and their relatives' experience of illness and medical treatment through anecdote in the home, at work and in the pub. These stories may be one of the major means by which people decide whether or not they should visit the doctor with their problem.[17]

A visit to the GP, or even more to the hospital clinic, is an important event which is frequently conveyed by anecdote to family and friends. It is at this stage that the understanding which the doctor thinks he or she has shared with the patient about the problem and its solution may go awry. The story of the visit is told and the listeners will comment on it, drawing upon their own experience and knowledge which is in turn often informed by anecdote. I overheard the following conversation whilst standing at a bus stop:

> Patient: The doctor told me I had high blood pressure and I've to start taking these tablets.
> Relative: Are you sure? I know Mr MacDonald down the road has got high blood pressure but he is twice the size of you and smokes like a chimney. He told me he had been getting terrible headaches and his doctor told him it was his blood pressure and he had to start cutting down. Perhaps you should just try cutting down a bit too.
> Patient: Yes. I don't feel unwell at all. I'll wait and see.

Media anecdotes

It is virtually impossible to open a newspaper without reading some kind of medical anecdote. Articles about the "bed crisis" in Britain's hospitals, for example, are frequently and aptly illustrated by a "trolley story" relating the experience of an (often) elderly patient who waited in a casualty cubicle for many hours, or an "ambulance story" about a cross-country mercy dash with a seriously ill patient in search of an intensive care bed. The dramatic experience of a sick individual sticks in the mind and may move people and politicians to action when dry facts and figures have failed.

Medical publications such as the *BMJ* and *BMA News Review* regularly publish accounts by patients of their experience of illness and medical treatment. Francine Stock, a BBC journalist, wrote about her experience of breast cancer in the BMA News Review and described the way her initial diagnosis was handled:

> A senior consultant was rushed in to do a biopsy. It would be fine, they chorused, crisis management was already in operation. The doctor could find a couple of lymph nodes but it would be fine – with a little chemotherapy, maybe a lumpectomy. Not to worry. All you need with cancer is a bit of luck, they said.[18]

The main function of such stories is probably to rouse doctors out of their complacency and make them realise how patients may see them.

Conclusion

As we have seen, anecdotes are an inevitable and essential part of communication within medicine and are in constant use between doctors, doctors and patients and in the lay community. They play many roles in these contexts but the important point is that by virtue of being dramatic, short and, therefore memorable, they have an impact upon the education of physicians, their understanding of patients' predicaments and even, occasionally, upon political decisions.

It is part of the art of medicine to be able to take all sources of information into account, to tap into many evidence sources, and through the art of clinical judgment, decide what is most relevant to the case in question. Clinical medicine deals with individuals, and the medical anecdote insists that attention focus upon the experience of the sick person.

--------------◄◊◊◊►--------------

1 Hunter KM. *Doctor's Stories: the narrative structure of medical knowledge.* Princeton: Princeton University Press, 1991, p. 71.
2 Mann RD. Breast implants: the tyranny of the anecdote. *J Clin Epidemiol* 1995; **48**: 504–6.
3 Macnaughton RJ. Anecdotes and empiricism. *Br J Gen Pract* 1995; **45**: 571-2.

4 *The Times* October 4 1997, p. 25.

5 Eraut M. *Developing professional knowledge and competence.* London: Falmer Press, 1994.

6 Schmidt HG, Norman GR, Boshuizen HPA. A cognitive perspective on medical expertise: theory and implications. *Academ Med* 1990; **65**: 611-21.

7 Sullivan FM, Macnaughton RJ. Evidence in consultations: interpreted and individualised. *Lancet* 1996; **348**: 941-3.

8 Tannenbaum S. What physicians know. *New Engl J Med* 1993; **329**: 1268-71.

9 See reference 1, p. 74.

10 Hunter KM. "There was this one guy...": the uses of anecdote in medicine. *Perspect Biol Med* 1986; **29**: 619-30.

11 Gillie A. The James Mackenzie Lecture : James Mackenzie and General Practice today. *The Practitioner* 1962; **188**: 94–107.

12 See reference 10, p. 621.

13 McBride WG. Thalidomide and congenital abnormalities. *Lancet* 1961; **ii**: 1358.

14 BMA and Royal Phamaceutical Society of Great Britain. *British National Formulary* **Number 34** (September 1997).

15 Guyatt G, Sackett D, Wayne Taylor D *et al.* Determining optimal therapy – randomised trials in individual patients. *New Engl J Med* 1986; **314**: 889–92.

16 Charlton B. Medical practice and the double-blind randomised controlled trial. *Br J Gen Pract* 1991; **41**: 355–6.

17 McKinlay JB. Social networks, lay consultation and help-seeking behaviour. *Social Forces* 1973; **51**: 275–92.

18 Stock F. My life in their hands: "I confronted cancer stormtrooper style". *BMA News Review* 1997; **23**: 50.

The Database of Individual Patient Experience

Trisha Greenhalgh

The Cochrane Collaboration is best known for its international endeavour to produce systematic reviews of all randomised controlled trials in the medical literature, and for its contribution to the theory and practice of meta-analysis (i.e. mathematical synthesis of the numerical results of clinical trials).[1] It publishes the Cochrane Library on CD ROM and the internet containing three widely used and continuously updated electronic databases of quantitative research – the Cochrane Controlled Trials Register (CCTR), the Cochrane Database of Systematic Reviews (CDSR), and the Database of Abstracts of Reviews of Effectiveness (DARE).

A new database, intended for use alongside the CDSR, the Database of Individual Patient Experience (DIPEX), is currently being developed. The aim of DIPEX will be to index, collate and publish in narrative form the illness experiences of health service users and participants in clinical trials. It is envisaged that DIPEX will eventually be accessed by patients, their families and carers, self help groups, policy makers, researchers, social scientists and medical and nursing educators as well as clinicians.

At the time of writing, the core team of six researchers, based in Oxford, UK, and led by Andrew Herxheimer and Anne McPherson, is preparing to undertake a systematic overview of the methods that have been used for collecting patients' illness experience in four clinical areas – breast cancer, pelvic pain, high blood pressure, and screening for bowel cancer. The DIPEX team plan to decide in the light of this review on the appropriate range of methods for compiling their database. They anticipate that a major contribution will come from reviews of the published literature and from new primary research in the form of semi-structured interviews.

The DIPEX team have analysed pilot questionnaires completed by patients after out-patient or in-patient hospital visits. These suggest that the final form for accounts on the DIPEX database will be as personal stories clearly anchored in relation to the diagnosis and stage of the patient's condition. Whenever possible, they will take a temporal perspective. Hence, rather than giving a single snapshot of the person's feelings and concerns at any one time during the course of an illness, the narrative will follow these feelings and concerns through a sequence that begins before the official diagnosis was made and continues through the clinical encounter, the investigations and management plan, and the resolution or progression of the disease.

Further information about the DIPEX project can be obtained from Pamela Baker, General Practice Research Group, Institute of Health Sciences, Headington, Oxford OX2 7LF, UK; Fax 01865 227 137; email pamela.baker@dphpc.ox.ac.uk

Acknowledgment

I am grateful to Dr Andrew Herxheimer, Emeritus Fellow, UK Cochrane Centre, for providing the information reproduced in this note.

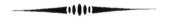

1 Chalmers I, Sackett D, Silagy C. The Cochrane Collaboration. In: Maynard A, Chalmers I eds *Non-random reflections on health services research*. London: BMJ Publishing Group, 1997, pp 231–9.

Broader perspectives on narrative in health care

21 Narrative in medical ethics

Anne Hudson Jones

Although narrative has always been important to medical ethics, only in the past two decades have literary scholars, ethicists, and health care professionals focused their attention directly on its role. The contributions of narrative to medical ethics come primarily in two ways: first, from the use of stories (narratives) for their *mimetic* content – that is, for what they say; and, second, from the methods of literary criticism and narrative theory for their analysis of *diegetic* form – that is, for their understanding of how stories are told and why it matters. Although narrative and narrative theory, like the form and content of a literary work, are inextricably bound up with each other, I will discuss them separately to help chart the evolving appreciation for the importance of narrative in the work of medical ethics.

The use of stories

During the past two decades, stories have been important to medical ethics in at least three major ways: first, as case examples for the teaching of principle based professional ethics, which has been the dominant form of medical ethics in the Western world; second, as moral guides to living a good life, not just in the practice of medicine but in all aspects of one's life; and, third, as narratives of witness that, with their experiential truth and passion, compel re-examination of accepted medical practices and ethical precepts.

Stories as cases for teaching principle based medical ethics

When medical humanities programmes were first being established in American medical schools in the 1970s and 1980s, historians, ethicists, and lawyers usually preceded scholars of literature on the faculty. The presence of historians can be explained by medicine's longstanding interest in its history; that of ethicists and lawyers, by the relevance of ethics and law to the problems of contemporary medical practice. A need for literary scholars was not self-evident: by 1982, only three medical schools in the US had a full-time professor of literature on the faculty.[1] In those early years, the presence of literature in medical humanities programmes was often justified by its service in the teaching of medical ethics.[2] Literary stories were found to be useful in "fleshing out" issues or dilemmas of medical ethics by showing them embedded in a particularized human context complicated by powerful emotions and complex interpersonal dynamics. Works by physician-writers have become staples of such teaching, and the short stories of William Carlos Williams[3] and Richard Selzer[4] have become especially well-known and frequently taught.

Narrated retrospectively from the physician's point of view, stories such as Williams' famous "The Use of Force"[5] and Selzer's "Brute"[6] offer insight into why a presumably good doctor with beneficent intentions nonetheless ends up harming his patient in an abuse of power. The first uses of these stories as cases for medical ethics may well have been limited to discussions of standard ethical principles such as autonomy or respect for persons, beneficence and non-maleficence, and social justice.[7] In principle based ethics, or principlism as it is sometimes called, general ethical principles are applied in a deductive analysis of a case to determine logically the best ethical resolution of its issues or dilemmas.[8] In both "The Use of Force" and "Brute", a physician physically assaults a patient in order to diagnose or treat. The ethical issue is whether such powerful medical paternalism can be justified by appealing to beneficence – that is, by claiming that what the physician did was for the patient's own good. But by attending to the richly evocative language used by the physician-narrators of these stories, readers have the opportunity to learn about more than patient autonomy and physician paternalism. They can learn how ethical principles and arguments may sometimes be used to rationalize unethical behavior that is driven by sexual attraction, anger, or pride.[9-11]

Although still controversial,[12-14] the use of such stories as literary cases to complement the teaching of principlism is the most basic way in which narrative has been important to medical ethics.

Narratives as moral guides for living a good life

The second way in which literary narratives have been important to medical ethics is best articulated by Robert Coles in his article "Medical Ethics and Living a Life".[15] Coles is concerned with moral inquiry of a far-ranging kind that does not limit itself to the practice of medicine. He is concerned with what it means to live a good life and, coincidentally, to practise medicine. Not professional medical ethics but existential ethics or virtue ethics is what he seeks to develop in his medical students. For this purpose, Coles believes that reading novels such as George Eliot's *Middlemarch,* Sinclair Lewis' *Arrowsmith,* F. Scott Fitzgerald's *Tender Is the Night,* and Walker Percy's *Love in the Ruins* works better than studying analytic ethics.

Although Coles chooses more complex literary texts than the short stories that are so often used as cases for the teaching of medical ethics, he chooses novels whose main characters are physicians. That is to say, the novels that he chooses take the world of medical practice as part of their subject matter. Yet narratives that serve as moral guides for living a good life need not be topically about medicine, as Anne Hunsaker Hawkins has argued in describing her use of Dante's *The Divine Comedy* with medical students.[16] From this larger perspective, any narrative that might instigate moral reflection about what it means to be a good person, to live a good life, and to practise a profession in an ethical manner could be considered important to medical ethics.

Narratives of witness

Autobiographical accounts by patients or by their family members or friends can also be important for medical ethics.[17] These works may not be as well written as those by established literary authors, but they can have considerable value as narratives of witness. Some of these narratives offer commentary from the patient's point of view on such ethical issues as autonomy and respect for persons, truth telling and informed consent, beneficence and, sometimes, maleficence – physicians' negligence, incompetence, and errors. As these narratives have begun to appear on the internet, they reach larger audiences and have the potential for more influence on the practices of particular physicians and institutions.[18] The implications of these electronic narratives for medical ethics are just beginning to be explored, but some physicians have incorrectly alleged that they constitute a violation of physician–patient confidentiality.[19] Physicians are ethically bound to maintain confidentiality about their patients, but patients are not similarly bound to maintain confidentiality about their physicians.

Patients and their family members and friends are not the only ones who write important narratives of witness. By writing narratives from their personal experiences, physicians and other health care professionals can also have a powerful effect on the public discussion of an ethical issue. In the US, for example, it was physicians' narratives of assisting patients' suicides that broke through decades of professional silence and opened debate about this issue in American medical journals. In 1982, after Richard Selzer published his fictional story "Mercy",[20] about a physician's unsuccessful attempt to help a terminally ill patient die by giving him an overdose of morphine, he received hate mail. A few years later, when the *Journal of the American Medical Association (JAMA)* published "It's over, Debbie",[21] an anonymous, presumably factual account by a physician who had deliberately given a terminally ill cancer patient an overdose of pain medication to speed her death, Cook County State's Attorney took the journal's editor to court to try to force him to reveal the author's identity. The effort was unsuccessful. And a few years later, after Timothy Quill published an eloquently written account of prescribing drugs for a patient who, he knew, intended to use them to commit suicide,[22] he was brought before a grand jury but was not indicted. Despite the general legal prohibition against physician-assisted suicide in the US, exemplified by the legal actions against *JAMA* and Quill, doctors' narratives have helped compel re-examination of this controversial ethical issue.

The methods of literary criticism and narrative theory

In the past decade, scholars have begun to use the methods of literary criticism and narrative theory to examine the texts and practices of traditional medical ethics. What are now referred to as *narrative approaches to medical ethics* or *narrative contributions to medical ethics* use techniques of literary analysis to enhance the practice of principle based medical ethics. In contrast, what has become known as *narrative ethics* has reconceptualized the practice of medical ethics, seeking to replace principlism with a paradigmatically different practice.

Narrative approaches to medical ethics

In those early years of medical humanities programmes in the US, the presence of literature was justified either on the basis of its service to medical ethics[2] or on the basis of claims that reading literature helps teach students "to read in the fullest sense",[23] a skill that helps prepare them for the clinical work of listening to and interpreting patients' stories,[24] as well as reconfiguring and retelling those stories as medical cases with plot and causality.[25] To read in the fullest sense, students must have mastered certain basic skills of literary analysis. The same questions that they learned to ask about a literary text – such questions as "Who is the narrator?", "Is the narrator reliable?", "From what angle of vision does the narrator tell the story?", "What has been left out of the narrative?", "Whose voice is not being heard and why?", "What kind of language and images does the narrator use?", and "What effect does that kind of language have in creating patterns of meaning that emerge from the text?" can also be used in the examination of ethical texts and practices.

One of the best examples of applying these methods to ethical texts is Tod S Chambers' work examining the inherent value biases in the ways that ethicists construct their cases.[26] Chambers shows that from their very first choices – point of view, diction, images, and other features of style – ethicists construct cases that lead readers to the conclusions which emanate from the author's ethical theories and preferences.

Rita Charon is the best known advocate of using the methods of literary criticism and narrative theory to help physicians and ethicists examine their ethical practices. The title of her article "Narrative contributions to medical ethics: recognition, formulation, interpretation, and validation in the practice of medical ethics" is in itself almost an abstract of the article and a summary of her position.[27] Making physicians and ethicists more aware of the narrative aspects of their medical and ethical practice will make them better physicians and ethicists, she argues. She hopes that narratively competent practitioners will actually be able to prevent ethical dilemmas from arising, by having conversations about ethics and values with their patients before a medical crisis throws them into an unanticipated ethical dilemma.

Narrative ethics

Kathryn Montgomery Hunter's work on the narrative structure of medical knowledge has helped clarify some of the mental processes that are involved in medical education and practice.[25] Unlike analytic philosophers who are trained to work deductively from general principles to the particular case, doctors are trained to work in the opposite direction, beginning with the particular case and then seeking general medical principles that might apply. Hunter argues that this practice is not inductive but abductive,[25 28 29] as doctors tack back and forth between the particular case and the generalized realm of scientific knowledge (see Chapter 24). This process is similar to that in the ethical practice of casuistry, which was revived and rehabilitated in an influential book by Jonsen and Toulmin.[30] In casuistry, ethical examination begins with the features of a particular case, then seeks to recall similar paradigm cases that may shed enlightenment about the best resolution for the case at hand (see Chapter 23). The similarity of mental process in medical thinking and casuistical thinking makes doctors better prepared by their training and practice to engage in casuistry than in the deductive process required in analytic principlism.[29] Casuistry is, arguably, one form of narrative ethics.

But narrative ethics has underlying assumptions that casuistry does not share. Foremost among them is a focus on the patient as narrator of his or her own story, including the ethical choices that belong to that story. Howard Brody has described a narrative ethics in which the physician must work as co-author with the patient to construct a joint narrative of illness and medical care.[31] This co-authoring involves more than simply recognizing the patient's autonomy as author. Brody calls it a relational ethic.[31] Arthur Kleinman and Arthur Frank have written about it from differing perspectives, the physician's and the patient's,[32 33] but both agree that such a narrative practice is relational and requires the physician to be an empathic witness of the patient's suffering.

In ideal form, narrative ethics recognizes the primacy of the patient's story[34] but encourages multiple voices to be heard and multiple stories to be brought forth by all those whose lives will be involved in the resolution of a case.[35 36] Patient, physician, family, nurse, friend, and social worker, for example, may all share their stories in a dialogical chorus[37] that can offer the best chance of respecting all the persons involved in a case.[38]

One reason narrative ethics is controversial and strongly opposed by some analytic philosophers may be that they may not themselves have the narrative skills necessary to listen to many voices, select significant details that cohere in patterns of meaning, and work toward resolutions arising from something other than logical, deductive processes.[39] That non-ethicists might have imaginative moral capacities that allow them to resolve ethical issues through a non-deductive process may be threatening to those who are accustomed to being in charge of ethical analysis. To move narrative ethics into a next phase of development, then, proponents must determine how training for competence in narrative ethics might best be achieved.[40] Reading and interpreting complex written narratives certainly helps, and that is part of what literature and medicine has been doing for 25 years now.[41] But for those whose professional training has not included such experiences, a kind of continuing education model that focuses on specific narrative skills may be helpful. Whether or not attaining greater narrative competence would make analytically trained ethicists more open to the possibilities of narrative ethics remains to be seen, but such training will do them no harm and it may lead to richer ethical discourse for us all.

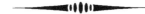

1 Trautmann J. Can we resurrect Apollo? *Literature and Medicine* 1982; **1**: 1–17.

2 Jones AH. Literature and medicine: traditions and innovations. In: Clarke B Aycock W eds. *The body and the text: comparative essays in literature and medicine.* Lubbock: Texas Tech University Press, 1990, pp. 11–24.

3 Williams WC. *The doctor stories.* Coles R (comp). New York: New Directions, 1984.

4 Selzer R. *Letters to a young doctor.* New York: Simon and Schuster/Touchstone Books, 1982.

5 Williams WC. The use of force. In: Williams WC. *The doctor stories.* Coles R (comp). New York: New Directions, 1984, pp. 56–60.

6 Selzer R. Brute. In: Selzer R. *Letters to a young doctor.* New York: Simon and Schuster/Touchstone Books, 1982, pp. 59–63.

7 Bell BC. Williams' "The use of force" and first principles in medical ethics. *Literature and Medicine* 1984; **3**: 143–51.

8 Beauchamp TL, Childress JL. *Principles of biomedical ethics*, 4th edition. New York: Oxford University Press, 1994.

9 Woodcock JA. Did Williams' doctor do the right thing? A disagreement between female and male medical students over "The use of force". *J Med Hum* 1992; **13**: 157–62.

10 King NMP, Stanford AF. Patient stories, doctor stories, and true stories: A cautionary reading. *Lit Med* 1992; **11**: 185–99.

11 Coles R. Introduction. In: Williams WC. *The doctor stories.* Coles R (comp). New York: New Directions, 1984, pp. vii–xvi.

12 Terry JS, Williams PC. Literature and bioethics: The tension in goals and styles. *Lit Med* 1988; **7**: 1–21.

13 Nelson HL ed. *Stories and their limits: narrative approaches to bioethics.* New York: Routledge, 1997.

14 Pickering N. Imaginary restrictions. *J Med Ethics* 1998; **24**: 171–5.

15 Coles R. Medical ethics and living a life. *N Engl J Med* 1979; **301**: 444–6.

16 Hawkins AH. Charting Dante: The *Inferno* and medical education. *Lit Med* 1992; **11**: 200–15.

17 Tovey P. Narrative and knowledge development in medical ethics. *J Med Ethics* 1998; **24**:176–81.

18 McLellan MF. The electronic narrative of illness. PhD dissertation. University of Texas Medical Branch, 1997.

19 Bulkeley WM. E-mail medicine: Untested treatments, cures find stronghold on on-line services. Doctors fret the gravely ill may share information and skew drug testing. No miracles from Neurontin. *Wall Street J*, February 27, 1995, pp. A1, A7A.

20 Selzer R. Mercy. In: Selzer R. *Letters to a young doctor.* New York: Simon and Schuster/Touchstone Books, 1982, pp. 70–4.

21 Anonymous. A piece of my mind. It's over, Debbie. *J Am Med Assoc* 1988; **259**(2): 272.

22 Quill TE. Death and dignity: a case of individualized decision making. *N Engl J Med* 1991; **324**: 691–4.

23 Trautmann J. The wonders of literature in medical education. In: Self DJ ed. *The role of the humanities in medical education.* Norfolk, VA: Teagle and Little, 1978, pp. 32–44.

24 Charon R. Doctor–patient/reader–writer: Learning to find the text. *Soundings* 1989; **72**: 137–52.

25 Hunter KM. *Doctors' stories: The narrative structure of medical knowledge.* Princeton, NJ: Princeton University Press, 1991.

26 Chambers TS. The bioethicist as author: the medical ethics case as rhetorical device. *Lit Med* 1994; **13**: 60–78.

27 Charon R. Narrative contributions to medical ethics: Recognition, formulation, interpretation, and validation in the practice of the ethicist. In: DuBose ER, Hamel RP, O'Connell LJ eds. *A matter of principles? Ferment in U.S. bioethics.* Valley Forge: Trinity Press International, 1994, pp. 260–83.

28 Eco U, Sebeok TA. *The sign of three: Dupin, Holmes, Peirce.* Bloomington: Indiana University Press, 1988.

29 Jones AH. Literature and medicine: narrative ethics. *Lancet* 1997; **349**: 1243–6.

30 Jonsen AR, Toulmin S. *The abuse of casuistry: a history of moral reasoning.* Berkeley: University of California Press, 1988.

31 Brody H. "My story is broken; can you help me fix it?" Medical ethics and the joint construction of narrative. *Lit Med* 1994; **13**: 79–92.

32 Kleinman A. *The illness narratives: suffering, healing, and the human condition.* New York: Basic Books, 1988.

33 Frank AW. *The wounded storyteller: body, illness, and ethics.* Chicago: University of Chicago Press, 1995.

34 Churchill LR. The human experience of dying: The moral primacy of stories over stages. *Soundings* 1979; **62**: 24–37.

35 Jones AH. Darren's case: narrative ethics in Perri Klass's *Other Women's Children. J Med Philos* 1996; **21**: 267–86.

36 Jones AH. From principles to reflective practice or narrative ethics? In: Carson RA, Burns CR eds. *Philosophy of medicine and bioethics: a twenty-year retrospective and critical appraisal.* Dordrecht: Kluwer Academic Publishers, 1997, pp. 193–5.

37 Bakhtin MM. *The dialogic imagination: four essays.* Holquist M ed. Emerson C, Holquist M (trans). Austin: University of Texas Press, 1981.

38 Best, PC. Making hospice work: collaborative storytelling in family-care conferences. *Lit Med* 1994: **13**: 93–123.

39 Clouser KD. Philosophy, literature, and ethics: Let the engagement begin. *J Med Philos* 1996; **21**: 321–40.

40 Jones AH. The color of the wallpaper: Training for narrative ethics. *HEC Forum* 1998; in press.

41 Charon R, Banks JT, Connelly JE *et al.* Literature and medicine: contributions to clinical practice. *Ann Intern Med* 1995; **122**: 599–606.

22 Anthropology and narrative

Vieda Skultans

> The sick woman lies in the hammock in front of you.
> Her white tissue lies in her lap, her white tissues move softly.
> The sick woman's body lies weak.
> When they light up along Muu*'s way, it runs over with exudations and like blood.
> Her exudations drip down below the hammock all like blood, all red.
> The inner white tissue extends to the bosom of the earth.
> Into the middle of the woman's white tissue a human being descends.[1]

The scope of medical anthropology

Levi-Strauss's classic account of Cuna shamanistic healing illustrates a number of important principles of medical anthropology. The song of the shaman (healer) is used to facilitate difficult childbirth. It translates the passage of the child from the womb through the birth canal as a quest in the Cuna; a place in popular myth peopled by spiritual entities. Through song the interior of the woman's body becomes inhabited by mythical beings and animals.[1]

Individual illness experience is profoundly influenced by society's perceptions and explanations of the meaning of illness and the mechanism of healing. Health professionals increasingly seek to understand the underlying cultural basis for differences in symptoms, illness behaviour and response to treatment that are known to exist across different cultural groups.

The Cuna song begins with an acknowledgment of the circumstances of the woman in labour and moves on to provide a spiritual and metaphysical frame for the physiological events. The shaman's song accords with the woman's own experience of labour,

* Muu is the power responsible for the formation of the fetus.

225

and contrasts with the sharp discrepancies between medical and lay illness narratives typical of Western medicine. The woman in labour is offered a language in which she can address her pain: "The cure would consist, therefore, in making explicit a situation originally existing on the emotional level and rendering acceptable to the mind pains which the body refuses to tolerate"[1] (p197).

This example shows that the illness narrative of a patient tells at least two stories: the highly personal experience of the illness itself, embedded within a deeper narrative of social networks, folk models, mythology and cultural history. This second, cultural narrative may itself contain a story of society's struggle for health and wholeness in an alien world. Accounts from a migrant or colonised culture, for example, often describe a shared past or present experience of separation, loss, physical hardship, discrimination, poverty, and persecution, all of which may be crucially important influences upon the nature and course of the illness. As we shall see, they may also offer a collective response to the experience of suffering.

The history of narrative analysis in anthropology

Anthropology has been shaped by empirical methods, particularly the fieldwork tradition of participant observation. Somewhat paradoxically, however, the informant's voice has often had to struggle to be heard in accounts that have tended to focus on theoretical and abstracted aspects of the work. Sperber expresses this through his imaginary heretic when he asks: "But was it necessary that the least academic form of research should yield the most academic form of literature?".[2] The roots of this unfortunate paradox can be traced all the way back to Plato, who explicitly devalued the expression of experience through art compared with the supposedly higher medium of theoretical discourse.

Plato's value system continues to influence modern studies where the anthropologist was present in the field but appears to be absent in the text. The fieldwork is reported through indirect speech, and the author's voice takes precedence over that of the actor. Even Kleinmann, in his polemic work of medical anthropology *The Illness Narratives*[3] tends to paraphrase the patients' stories and in the process filter them through the prism of psychiatric history taking.

However, the relatively recent tradition of recording and analysing narrative and life stories is at last becoming respectable in anthropological circles. In the 1950s and 1960s, such fieldwork tended to be done by women while their partners engaged in the "serious work" of collecting ethnographic data.[4] Laura Bohannen's autobiographical account of collecting life stories in *Return to Laughter* is an example of just such a division of labour; it was published under the pseudonym of Elenore Smith Bowen and proclaimed itself as fiction.[5]

But more recent works have upheld the validity of authentic narrative over the anthropologist's representation and translation.[6] Language comes saturated with earlier meanings derived from other contexts of use. Language absorbs shared meanings and values: it comes in pre-assembled parts;[7] hence, it conveys truths both about primary level culture (the underlying beliefs and value systems that determine observed behaviour) and about the relationship between the ethnographer and his or her informants.[8]

As Glyn Elwyn and Richard Gwyn show in Chapter 17, such truths are often deep seated and may become apparent only after sophisticated analysis of the text. Fluency in the language is, therefore, a precondition for working with narratives. We would now probably interpret Evans-Pritchard's dismissal of the services of his Nuer interpreter a few months after his arrival in Nuerland as naïve and a major deficiency in his approach to fieldwork.[9]

In the early years of narrative analysis in anthropology, the analysis of direct speech was used primarily to access aspects of culture which were considered otherwise impenetrable. The worlds of prostitution, crime and drug dealing were unlocked through the recording of individual life stories. More recent theoretical work on the use of narrative in cultural analysis no longer assumes recorded speech to be an unproblematic conduit to reality. Indeed, part of the fascination in authentic narrative lies in its ambivalence. It does not simply reach out to some external truth but, in the attempt to describe reality, it constructs experience and identity and even, at times, creates a fictional or mythical reality (see, for example, Shirley Brice Heath[10] for an account of the different uses of language in the Piedmont Carolinas, and Labov[11][12] for an analysis of the dramatic structure of the language of the inner city).

Illness as crisis; narrative as hope

Narratives play a particularly important role where there is a breach between the ideal and the real.[13] Crises feed the narrative drive. Thus, illness comes to have a particularly close relationship with narrative. Illnesses acquire a moral meaning through plot, through embeddedness in a life story, and, conversely, the individual illness experience serves as a wider metaphor for the suffering society. Narrative introduces new possibilities in a life narrowed down by illness. Byron Good uses the term *subjunctivisation* to convey the way in which narrativisation opens up possibilities of alternative life trajectories in chronic disability.[14] [15] Frank writes of the diseased body's need for a voice and outlines for us the principal plots of Western illness narratives: the restitution, the quest, the chaos and the testimonial narratives.[16]

The existence of such plots underlines the fact that the most personal of recollections are shaped by existing genres of story telling in a society. Our experiences may be personal but their transposition into stories must have shared elements in order to be intelligible. The extent to which the health professional can recognise this social dimension of story-telling is probably the extent to which he or she is sensitive to the cultural differences in the experience of illness and the meanings accorded to it. Our own paradigmatic illness stories, used in the context of health education or attempts at empathy, may therefore have no meaning for patients from other cultures.

Illness narratives as cultural history

Narrative is closely linked to memory. Memory is selective and its principles of selection are shaped by social forces. Halbwachs, an early pioneer in the study of social memory, said:

> Our memories remain collective … and are recalled to us through others even though only we were participants in the events or saw the things concerned. In reality we are never alone. Other men need not be physically present, since we always carry within us and in us a number of distinct persons.[17]

Tonkin describes narratives of the past as constituting a genre: "a mode or code for people's transmission of experience, and, as well, by its own transmission, maintains a version of the past that people can use for their own ends".[18]

My own recent work on neurasthenia in Latvia has sought to understand biographical accounts of illness in terms of their historical and socio-political setting.[19] [20] The paradigms of illness story-telling discussed by Frank (restitution, quest, chaos and testimonial) are, in this context, replaced with an account of a shared oppression and collective destiny.

> Working in the forest I fell ill with acute pneumonia and afterwards with bronchial asthma. The illness got worse in winter, I couldn't do anything outside, I couldn't accompany the children to their school 7 kilometres away. I didn't dare get hot preparing food, washing clothes, because after that there would be acute attacks. It was very difficult to breathe, with every movement it got worse – I was suffocating, my lungs creaked, I could not draw the air in. ... One lived a solitary life because the nearest neighbours had been deported, other houses were far away and in the winter there were no roads around our house. Husband to work, schoolboy to school, trudging on foot or on skis. It was a problem to bring the doctor home, because the supervisor was unwilling to release my husband from work. In that fashion I was ill for 18 years. In between attacks I went to several doctors in the regional polyclinic to the doctors in the neighbouring village clinic. But such journeys often ended sadly. Buses were a long way away (7 kilometres) the better doctors 20 kilometres away. The journey, the long wait in the overfilled waiting rooms would trigger off a new attack, but not of course straight away. ... The simpler injections in the muscle my husband injected or I myself. I treated myself with bees venom – getting the bees to sting me. I started with a smaller number and increased the number every day. All according to the doctor's instructions. I use herbal teas a lot.
>
> In the hospital where our village had to be treated, the doctors viewed people of working age as simulants (malingerers) who did not want to work and expected to be fed in hospital and they said so openly – "I don't know what you want from hospital" and so on ... I very much wanted to be cured but came up against suspicion, all the family members suffered, because they were always reminded of my not working in a waged capacity. With great effort, even writing to the Ministry of Health I succeeded in being issued with a temporary medical certificate that I was not able to work in damp and cold weather and that I was not able to do heavy work.
>
> *Mara, a Latvian countrywoman from Vidzeme*

The narrative is, of course, about a personal experience of illness. But that experience is shaped by a shared cultural lens which puts the illness to critical use. Latvian illness narratives constitute a distinctive genre of social criticism. Latvian understandings of illness causation, of its development and exacerbation over time, of treatment or failures of treatment and the personal consequences and family ramifications of illness are tightly interwoven with the perceived shortcomings of the Soviet regime in post-war Latvia. Indeed, Mara's account moves outwards from the actual illness experience to the society in which she lived. In the process of this social embedding she gives us not only a medical but a social history. We are given a graphic description of inadequately treated asthma, but we also learn about compulsory forest work, the expropriation of peasant land, deportations, the depopulation of the countryside, extreme poverty and lack of basic amenities. Although this is a deeply felt and unique life history, Mara's narrative also belongs to a distinctive genre of Latvian story-telling in which illness is perceived as having its roots in the inhumane and contradictory expectations of Soviet society. It thereby provides a tool for criticising that society but also enables narrators to link their lives and suffering with those of countless others.

Whose story?

A central question in medical anthropology is: who has the authority to tell the story of the sick person? In many cross-cultural situations, the sickness story belongs to either the medical attendant or the lay carers, but not to the sick person themselves. Basil Sansom who worked among Aborigines in Darwin recorded that in this society, "You caan [can't] tell about that time you bin sick".[21] Rather, the sick role and its requirements create the "perpetuation of relationships of long-term indebtedness amongst a community of people who have no property but rely instead on verbal warranties" (p. 183). Thus, those who help the sick may tell the story of the illness, and in the telling, they both describe and create the social network that allows the illness to be attended:

> Tommy Atkins' cough, said Bill, was due to strychnine. Years ago down on the droving trail, Big Bill, Tommy Atkins and four named others set out to collect a mob of cattle to herd over towards Tennant Creek. When night fell, they camped at a site near a billabong. Other campers had been there before them and the previous occupants had left behind some strong quart size tin cans, empty and very shiny. Tommy Atkins said that was good. He twisted fencing wire to give one of the tins a handle and so turn it into a billy can. He set water to boil as did the others. On the fire the new can kept company with five soot-encrusted billies. After drinking his tea, Tommy was

seized with convulsions. As Big Bill explained, the tin had
been used by men who were after the dingo bounty. It had
held poison for making dingo baits.

The remainder of the story is a detailed account of the rescue of
Tommy Atkins through the communal effort of his colleagues.
Everyone did the right thing – made Tommy vomit, kept him
warm, tied him to a horse, ensured his timely arrival at the doctor's
surgery. The Drover saw the patient in his state of "very danger"
and was a member of a local community of concern made up of
people who "worried for" Tommy Atkins until he was declared to
be not "really sick" any more. When a recovered Tommy Atkins
returned to the camps, people watched him and sought to divine
what changes the ordeal had wrought in him (p. 186–7).

This extract again illustrates how illness stories tend to be
embedded in a specific locality and a web of social relationships,
which are drawn out in the description of how the illness is
managed. Janzen's work in Zaire also showed the importance of
what he called the therapy management group for articulating the
illness story and deciding upon appropriate courses of treatment.[22]

Their work highlights the importance of identifying the source of
illness narratives. Whose voice has the right to be heard and how
are contested issues decided? The example of Tommy Atkins is
relatively unproblematic in that he belongs to a culture in which
illness imposes silence on the sufferer. In other cultures, the
Western medical culture included, where there is less consensus,
different voices vie to be heard. For example, Rob Barrett, who is
both a psychiatrist and an anthropologist, gives us a brilliant
analysis of the way in which narratives of psychiatric cases
incorporate the different voices of the psychiatric team. The case
study is a "segmented object" which reflects the schisms within the
psychiatric hospital.[23] The different segments of the case study
reflect the distinctive voices of the nursing staff, the social workers
and the psychiatrists. As the team leader the psychiatrist had the
authority to integrate these distinctive voices into a single
narrative.

One of the most interesting recent developments in the science
of narrative analysis in anthropology is the analysis of self
awareness or reflexivity, which draws on the work of literary
theorists such as Wolfgang Iser[24] and social psychologists such as
Jerome Bruner,[25] John Shotter,[26] and Kenneth and Mary Gergen.[27]

Awareness of one's own story, one's own part in a dialogue, has as a necessary corollary the recognition of the voice of the other. The dichotomy between researcher and human being which Elizabeth Bowen sought to emphasize in the preface of *Return to Laughter* can no longer be upheld. There, reflecting a now outdated dualism, she wrote: "When I write as a social anthropologist and within the canons of that discipline, I write under another name. Here I have written simply as a human being, and the truth I have tried to tell concerns the sea change in one's self that comes from immersion in another and alien world."[5] The many ambiguities of the narrative "I", referring as it does both to the author of a text, the voice of the narrator and to the actor at different stages of the life course all come to be subjected to detailed scrutiny in the course of narrative analysis.

The reflective, first-person narrative gives a unique insight into the experience of illness. Illness entails changes that call out for explanation. Everyday routines and relationships, hitherto taken for granted, are disrupted, and expectations can no longer be met. Sometimes these changes require a fundamental reconstruction of one's sense of self and identity. Narrative is the means by which such changes can be brought about, since personally constructed stories about self provide a space in which values can be reasserted and new roles described. The stories tell us not simply what has happened, but what kind of person the narrator is. In becoming the author of a new life story, the sick person becomes able to take control of the new situation.

Narratives facilitate the search for, and construction of, new meanings in situations where the old meanings no longer work. They do not, however, mirror past events in a straightforward way. Because, as Kierkegaard reminds us, we live our lives forward but understand them backwards, our narrative understandings are not fixed in stone. They are fluid, ever changing entities in which the present and the past and the individual narrator and their culture are in a perpetual state of interplay. Narrative understanding is thus not only a challenge for anthropology but a key to understanding oneself and others.

---

1 Levi-Strauss C. *Structural Anthropology.* New York: Basic Books, 1963.
2 Sperber D. *On Anthropological Knowledge.* Cambridge: Cambridge University Press, 1985, p. 7.

3 Kleinman A. *The Illness Narratives: Suffering, Healing and the Human Condition.* New York: Basic Books, 1988.

4 Langness LL. *The Life History in Anthropological Science.* New York: Holt, Rinehart and Winston, 1965, p. 20.

5 Bowen Smith E. *Return to Laughter.* London: Victor Gollancz, 1956.

6 Clifford J and Marcus GE eds. *Writing Culture. The Poetics and Politics of Ethnography.* Berkeley: University of California Press, 1986.

7 Smith Herrnstein B. *On the Margins of Discourse. The Relation of Literature to Language.* Chicago and London: University of Chicago Press, 1979.

8 Fabian J. *Time and the Other. How Anthropology Makes its Object.* New York: Columbia University Press, 1983.

9 Evans-Pritchard S. *The Nuer.* Oxford: Clarendon Press, 1940, p. 14.

10 Heath S Brice. *Ways with Words. Language, Life and Work in Communities and Classrooms.* Cambridge: Cambridge University Press, 1983.

11 Labov W. The Transformation of Experience in Narrative Syntax. In *Language in the Inner City.* Philadelphia: University of Pennsylvania Press, 1972, pp. 354–96.

12 Labov W, Waletzky J. Narrative Analysis: Oral Versions of Personal Experience. In: *Essays on the Verbal and Visual Arts. Proceedings of the 1966 Annual Spring Meeting of the American Ethnological Society.* Croom Helm, 1974.

13 Riessman C Kohler. *Narrative Analysis.* London: Sage Publications, 1993, p. 3.

14 Good BJ. *Medicine, Rationality and Experience. An Anthropological Perspective.* Cambridge: Cambridge University Press, 1994.

15 Good BJ, Good M-J DelVecchio. In the subjunctive mode: epilepsy narratives in Turkey. *Soc Sci Med* 1994; **38**: 835–42.

16 Frank AW. *The Wounded Storyteller. Body, Illness and Ethics.* Chicago: Chicago University Press, 1995.

17 Halbwachs M. *The Collective Memory.* New York: Harper and Row, 1981 (first published 1950), p. 23.

18 Tonkin E. *Narrating our Pasts. The Social Construction of Oral History.* Cambridge: Cambridge University Press, 1995, p. 114.

19 Skultans V. A historical disorder: neurasthenia and the testimony of lives. *Anthropol Med* 1997; **4**: 7–24.

20 Skultans V. *The Testimony of Lives. Narrative and Memory in Post-Soviet Latvia.* London: Routledge, 1997.

21 Sansom B. The Sick Who do not Speak. In: Parkin D ed. *Semantic Anthropology.* London: Academic Press, 1982, p. 184.

22 Janzen JM. *The Quest for Therapy in Lower Zaire.* Berkeley: University of California Press, 1978.

23 Barrett R. *The Psychiatric Team and the Social Definition of Schizophrenia. An Anthropological Study of Person and Illness.* Cambridge: Cambridge University Press, 1996, p. 39.

24 Iser W. *Prospecting. From Reader Response to Literary Anthropology.* Baltimore and London: John Hopkins University Press, 1989.

25 Bruner J. The Autobiographical Process. *Current Sociology* 1995; **43**: 161–77.

26 Shotter J, Gergen KJ eds. *Texts of Identity.* London: Sage Publications, 1989.

27 Gergen M, Gergen K. The Social Construction of Narrative Accounts. In: Gergen M and Gergen K eds. *Historical Social Psychology.* New Jersey and London: Erlbaum Associates, 1984, pp. 173–90.

23 The wounded storyteller:[1] narrative strands in medical negligence

Brian Hurwitz

> None of the doctors told me. I asked them what really
> happened to my baby … . I asked them crying and I asked
> them OK and I asked them mad. And they didn't tell me.[2]

Shivers run down medical spines and students look up and take
note at the very mention of negligence.[3] The term evokes vague
scenes of things going wrong, procedures that fail, of muddle,
misunderstanding, poor communication, and fear.

A leading lawyer's manual on how to conduct this kind of
litigation begins by evoking the atmosphere of a gothic novel:

> We love and fear doctors and particularly surgeons. Despite
> our era of tatty hospital corridors, technology and Trusts, a
> faint air of necromancy hangs around them still; there is a
> touch of the White Knight and there is a touch of the
> Magus.[4]

The scene here is reminiscent of *Doctor Jekyll and Mr Hyde*; the role
of the law (and its agents) is to impose vital checks upon the
dangerous effects of unbridled power visited by doctors upon
unwitting individuals already vulnerable from illness.

Patients sue doctors in the hope of gaining financial compensation for harm they have suffered during treatment. But a narrative
motive also animates claims: legal action may appear to offer the
best prospect of forcing a treatment story into the open, of telling
a tale of suffering or of dashed hopes, exploring where accountabil-
ity for injury lies, of gaining due recognition, achieving a dialogue
with medical staff, or extracting an apology.[5][6]

A narrative understanding of litigation illuminates how medicine and law interact, and suggests approaches to clinical work likely to minimise resort to legal action. A desire to be fully informed, to understand the nature of the medical narrative which has engulfed somebody's life, can be overwhelmingly strong, as Sandra Gilbert movingly portrays in writing about the death of her husband: "over and over again each of us murmurs the same refrain – 'What happened? What could have happened?' – as if these words were a talisman … 'What happened? What could have happened?' "[7] To know the reason *why*, and if no one knows why, then at least to determine (sometimes in minute detail) *how* events came to unfold this particular way, are the raw needs of many injured patients and their relatives. It is when such intensely felt human needs remain unmet that people are driven to seek legal redress.

What is negligence?

Defined in the Oxford English Dictionary as "a want of attention to what ought to be done", negligence always suggests a narrative context. A negligent action is one that fails to meet an expected and (by society's standards) achievable level of performance. Medical events unfolding in time according to impersonal causes and the best of human intentions may, in consequence, take a sinister turn.[8]

Several narrative strands can be seen interweaving in legal actions alleging medical negligence. To begin with, the injured patient's account (the plaintiff's version of events) jostles with the defendant doctor's narrative of what is thought to have happened. Initially, the contest is to establish a single story pieced together out of the telling, re-telling, revision and refashioning of memories; but from the outset, each party's memories are confronted with the sequence of events revealed by the medical records, tracings and the results of investigations – the "hard" record of what happened (see Chapter 19).

Every legal dispute is based upon facts, and "every legal mode of resolving those disputes involves a recounting and narrative refashioning of those facts".[9] No matter how strong a plaintiff's case may initially sound, the advice a plaintiff receives on whether to proceed with a claim, will be strongly influenced by the contemporaneous written medical record. The judicial process accords written records a privileged (though not an unchallengeable) position as evidence of what did, or did not, take place during treatment; and court cases may turn on whose narrative account the judge believes best matches the written record.

Before a dispute can come before a court for resolution a series of formal procedures has to be set in train. In the UK, a *Writ of Summons* must be served, which defines who the plaintiff(s) and defendant(s) are, and states the legal nature of the claim. The writ demands damages for personal injuries caused by the defendant's negligence, without necessarily defining any of the details as to what allegedly happened. Such details will be included in the plaintiff's *Statement of Claim*; this sets out the facts, and also details the allegation of negligence to which the defendant prepares a formal response on the basis of his or her version of events.

In cases involving allegations of medical negligence, the plaintiff's lawyers may well seek sight of hospital or other medical records before proceedings are commenced (to better evaluate a plaintiff's prospects of success). Once litigation has been started, proceedings will consist of activities which take place before trial – referred to as *interlocutory* steps – and the trial itself. *Interlocutory* steps commence with the Statement of Claim and the defendant's response. There follows a highly structured and ritualised series of written exchanges – referred to as the *Requests for Further and Better Particulars* and *Interrogatories* – in which each party's solicitors request clarification and expansion of the other side's case. At the same time, the process of discovery takes place, during which each side reveals further details of its own case, such as relevant records and written documentation. By the time any dispute comes to court, the details of the plaintiff's original claim, and the narrative which it recounts, may have been modified as a result.

Witness statements from bystanders to the relevant events are also exchanged, together with reports from expert witnesses commissioned to give their opinion about the perceived significance and reasonableness of the treatment that unfolded. During this process of refinement and adjustment of the claim and its detailed defence, some 50% or more of claims activated by patients are abandoned as unsustainable.[10]

In the courts, narratives of human lives intersect with those of medical careers within a syntax determined by legal structures. The law demands stereotypical roles (plaintiff/defendant), a chorus of supporting voices (expert witnesses) and a denouement (resolution imposed by judgment). Previously, medical negligence actions in the UK involved a court hearing in front of a jury. Today, however, these actions are resolved by a judicial process without a jury, though the jury has been retained in other jurisdictions, such as the USA. A court's fundamental task is to *hear* all the evidence, to reconstruct an official depiction of the events in question: "the facts". What happened, why did it happen, and (on the balance of probabilities) what were the consequences?

In 1956, Mr John Bolam claimed damages from Friern Hospital Management Committee in London, UK, for the electro-convulsive treatment (ECT) he received in 1954 for treatment of a severe episode of depression. He provided signed consent for the procedure, but he was not warned at the time of possible associated risks.

Neither Bolam nor his doctors knew that this event would give rise to a landmark legal case in the courts. In accordance with the normal practice at Friern, ECT was administered without applying any form of manual restraint other than supporting Mr Bolam's chin and holding down his shoulders. As a result of unrestrained muscular spasms provoked by ECT, he sustained "stove-in" fractures to both hips. These were the facts agreed by both parties to the dispute.

Mr Bolam contended that the Hospital Management Committee and its agents (the medical staff) had been negligent in administering ECT without using relaxant drugs or manually restraining his convulsive movements, and in failing to warn him of the risk he was taking in agreeing to undergo ECT. The Management Committee denied both these claims, maintaining that the treatment he received was not substandard but accorded with the standard of care to be expected (at that time) in these circumstances. Thus far, two different meanings had been attributed to a course of action composing a single narrative strand of events.

The case came to court in February 1957. Expert witnesses informed the court of the different techniques commonly adopted in administering ECT, including the use of either muscle relaxant drugs or strong manual restraint. The court was informed that the fracture rate associated with ECT was of the order of 1 in 10,000, and the judge reviewed Friern Hospital's fracture figures to see whether the rate had increased since adoption of manual restraint without relaxant drug administration.

Once "the facts" have been established, it is for the court to determine their *legal significance*. In narrative terms, the court's job is to write an official conclusion to the story it has heard. If the events that have been recounted meet various criteria demanded by UK common law and conform to a particular logical structure – the legal grammar of negligence actions – the plaintiff is likely to be successful, and damages awarded. But in order to qualify for formal decision making by legal process, the vernacular narrative of the plaintiff must first be remodelled by processes that bear comparison with the transformation of patients' narratives into medical case histories. Solicitors consulted by aggrieved patients must identify key elements from the story they hear. To prove negligence a plaintiff (the person bringing the action) must show that:

- the defendant doctor owed the plaintiff a *duty of care*;
- the doctor *breached* this duty of care by failing to provide the *required standard of medical care*;
- this failure actually *caused* the plaintiff harm.

The categories in this formulation have attained particular legal meanings arising from an evolving discourse fashioned from previous cases decided by the courts. Together with the narrative versions of events recounted by the opposing parties, this evolving legal discourse forms the dominant element in the narrative strands of medical negligence actions.

Duty of care

The common law holds that once a doctor–patient relationship exists, doctors have a *duty of care* towards their patients, the nature of which was spelt out in the UK in 1925, during a case involving a traumatic forceps delivery. The judge stated then that:

> If a person holds himself out as possessing special skill and knowledge, and he is consulted as possessing such skill and knowledge ... he owes a duty to the patient ... to use diligence, care, knowledge, skill and caution in administering treatment. No contractual relation is necessary, nor is it necessary that the service be rendered for reward.[11]

Thus defined, the doctor's duty of care is imposed by law; its standard in a particular case is determined by the courts after hearing expert evidence.

Reasonable standard

The standard of treatment a doctor owes to a patient derives from the decisions made in Bolam's case. In the oft repeated words of Mr Justice McNair in this case:

> ... where you get a situation which involves the use of some special skill or competence, then the test as to whether there has been negligence or not is not the test of the man on the top of the Clapham omnibus, because he has not got this special skill. The test is the standard of the ordinary skilled man exercising and professing to have that special skill. A man need not possess the highest expert skill; ... it is sufficient if he exercises the ordinary skill of an ordinary competent man exercising that particular art. A doctor will not be guilty of negligence if he has acted in accordance with a practice accepted as proper by a responsible body of medical men skilled in that particular art.[12]

This is what has become known as the "Bolam test". Expert testimony – the opinions of doctors in the field – helps the courts ascertain what is accepted and proper medical practice in specific cases; and this generally ensures that professionally generated clinical standards – rather than standards originating from elsewhere – are applied.[13][14]

Having listened to a number of expert witness accounts, the judge in the Bolam case concluded that at the time of John Bolam's treatment, competent doctors held divergent views both about the desirability of using relaxant drugs during ECT, and about the value of manual control of the patient. According to his judgment,

> ... a doctor is not negligent, if he is acting in accordance with such a practice, merely because there is a body of opinion that takes a contrary view ...[15]

The judge's formulations in Bolam have become the most influential statements of the standard of medical care required by UK law; and they still hold sway over how cases of medical negligence, particularly with respect to diagnosis and treatment, are decided in UK courts.

Causation

Successful negligence actions are fault based, i.e. the plaintiff must show, on the balance of probabilities, that the breach of duty *caused* or *materially contributed to* injury.[16] Lord Justice Denning formulated factual causation in this way:

> If the damage would not have happened but for a particular fault then the fault is the cause of the damage; if it would have happened just the same, fault or no fault, the fault is not the cause of the damage.[17]

In addition to proving causation in fact, causation in law requires also to be proved. This involves showing that the damage actually brought about by a particular act or omission was both foreseeable and reasonably avoidable.[18]

The case of *Early v Newham Health Authority* (1994) illustrates the operation of two of these concepts in the context of a story very different from that of John Bolam's. The plaintiff, a 13-year-old-girl, alleged that an anaesthetist had employed a faulty protocol during a failed intubation procedure.[19] Prior to elective surgery, it had proved impossible to pass an anaesthetic tube into the windpipe during an otherwise routine operation. The anaesthetist duly followed a protocol adopted in that hospital for such eventualities. This recommended insufflation of the lungs with an oxygen-rich mixture until the patient regained consciousness. During the course of the procedure the patient awoke whilst still paralysed from the anaesthetic, suffering fright and distress as a result.

The facts of the case were not disputed by the two parties. But in bringing the action, the plaintiff's *interpretation* of the agreed narrative was very different from that of the defendants'. Ms Early alleged that the protocol used in her care had been substandard; the defendants denied this.

The judge heard evidence about the origins of the protocol, its development and manner of adoption by the hospital's division of anaesthesia, and expert witnesses informed him of its use in other UK hospitals. He concluded that the authors of this protocol had been responsible and competent, and ruled that neither the doctor nor the health authority had been negligent in approving and adopting it.

Breach of duty

In the Early case there was no need formally to establish a duty of care between anaesthetist and patient because the existence of a relationship of reliance by the patient upon the reasonable skills of the anaesthetist was incontestable. The nub of the case turned on whether there had been a breach of duty, a failure by the doctor to provide the required standard of care. This was decided upon by the judge after evidence had been heard concerning the practices typically adopted by anaesthetists in clinical situations of this sort, and of the need to balance risks involved in alternative courses of action, such as the risk of transient terror if consciousness is regained, against the danger of prolonging anaesthesia by addition of an anaesthetic agent until paralysis has worn off.

Even had breach of duty been proven in a case such as Early, the action for negligence could in principle still have failed if the plaintiff could not also prove, on the balance of probabilities, that the breach of duty actually caused the injury complained of. In other words, had it been found that the anaesthetist had adopted a substandard protocol and was thereby in breach of his duty, the next question to be answered by a court would have been "did the plaintiff, on the balance of probabilities, suffer physical or psychological injury as a result?" If the answer to this question in such circumstances had been "yes", then the action would be successful and the defendants would be liable for damages. If the answer to this question had been "no" (almost inconceivable in a case such as Early) then despite the finding of a demonstrable breach of duty, the defendants would not be liable for any damages.

A court will endeavour to discern the paradigmatic elements to a dispute – the extent to which the case under consideration is similar to previously decided cases of alleged negligence. Abstracting and delineating the archetypal legal nature of each story, the material facts, is fundamental to this task. The court may then compare and distinguish various "plots" of previously decided actions and the legal principles underpinning their outcome.[20]

Variations upon a basic theme

Myriad possible plots can be based upon the "complex calculus" of negligence.[21] In 1953, a case turned upon whether the law recognises a duty upon doctors to be aware of recently published findings bearing upon the standard of care patients can expect from their doctor. In *Crawford v Board of Governors of Charing Cross Hospital* (1953) the plaintiff had been born with a useless left arm.[22] At the age of 52 he was admitted to hospital for a routine bladder operation. But because of the prolonged position in which his good arm had been placed during the operation (to allow free flow to an intravenous drip), he was left with severe nerve palsy resulting in a permanently useless right arm.

A lower court had found the anaesthetist to have been negligent. But this finding was later reversed by the Court of Appeal which noted that the shoulder had been maintained in the usual posture in accordance with customary practice at the time. In Lord Justice Somervell's view there was no evidence that the standard of care which Crawford received during the operation had departed from that which was customary at the time, and this excluded a finding of negligence.

In Somervell's view, the first judge had erred in basing his comments upon the anaesthetist's failure to read an article in *The Lancet* which had been published 6 months prior to the operation, pointing out the danger of brachial nerve palsy if an arm was kept in the postition concerned in Crawford's case for the period of time required by his operation. Lord Justice Denning concurred:

> It would, I think, be putting too high a burden on a medical man to say that he has to read every article appearing in the current medical press; and it would be quite wrong to suggest that the medical man is negligent because he does not at once put into operation the suggestion that some contributor or other might make in a medical journal. The time may come in a particular case when a new recommendation may be so well proved and so well known, and so well accepted that it should be adopted, but that was not so in this case.[23]

The legal auditorium

A related issue is raised by *Vernon v Bloomsbury Health Authority* (1995). The plaintiff, Barbara Vernon, was treated in hospital in 1982 for culture negative bacterial endocarditis. She had received doses of gentamicin higher than those recommended by the *Product Data Sheet*, the *British National Formulary* (*BNF*), the *Monthly Index of Medical Specialities* (*MIMS*) and *Martindale's Extra Pharmacopoeia*, and for a period longer than that recommended by *MIMS* and *Martindale*. She had been given 5.625 mg of the drug per kg of her body weight for 19 days, whereas these reference sources at the time recommended a maximum dose of 5 mg/kg for

7 days. As a consequence of this treatment, Barbara Vernon suffered damage to the balance apparatus of her inner ears.

At the hearing, all but one of the expert witnesses testified that they themselves would have prescribed gentamicin at this dosage for a patient in Barbara Vernon's condition. The plaintiff's expert witness stated that she would not herself have administered such a high dose for this condition, but she was unable to say that no reasonably competent microbiologist would have prescribed at this level. The judge found that:

> ... the dosage was a proper one. The doctors were not negligent in prescribing it. I agree with the defendants' experts that the guidelines laid down by the manufacturers and, for example, *MIMS*, are too conservative and that they err on the side of caution. I accept the views expressed by Dr Sowton, Dr Reeves and Dr Cooke, all of whom have great practical experience of prescribing this drug. In particular, I rely on the views of Dr Reeves. He has consistently prescribed higher doses than those recommended by the manufacturers and has advised others to do the same.[24]

This judgment highlights the extent to which, in fashioning legal conclusions to contested narratives, a court provides a controlled auditorium in which testimonies are heard, interrogated, tested and weighed.[25] Once a court has handed down judgment, the narrative which brought both parties to the legal auditorium is officially at a close, its legally fashioned conclusion awaiting official inscription in the annals of society's civil narratives.[26]

Untold stories

The legal narratives described here are stories without endings. We do not know, and we shall probably never know, what became of Bolam, Early, Crawford, and Vernon in the world beyond the courtroom. Bolam's name continues to reverberate in legal rulings, since the judgment in his case formulated important legal principles. His name has come to be repeated endlessly: in judgments, case reports, textbooks, jurisprudential comment, indices, and legal databases; and it appears, also, on many of the official policy documents of health care organisations, and in risk management manuals. In this sense Bolam's story lives on, as part of a larger legal narrative, touching upon the mishaps and misfortunes of many others. Though they returned a verdict for the defendants, the jury in his case expressed their sympathies to Mr Bolam for the terrible injuries he had received, and conveyed the hope that he would find some organisation to help alleviate his position.

The tragedy that awaits the completion of a court's consideration of medical negligence arises from the dichotomous result that necessarily ensues: compensation for the injured patient and disgrace (even ignominy) for the doctor, or nothing for the patient and total exoneration of the doctor. All four of the actions discussed in this chapter failed. Compared with the 85% success rate for UK personal injury claims in non-medical contexts, only 17% of cases which allege medical negligence in the UK succeed.[27] A number of possible reasons for this disparity have been put forward; some actions are brought inappropriately, whilst others are settled out of court;[28] and many cases which stand a good chance of success are never begun.[29] This combination of factors is responsible for a hidden malpractice denominator.[30–32]

The chances of winning legal actions of this class, once they come to court, remain strongly in the defendants' favour, partly as a result of the hidden denominator, and partly because many indefensible claims are settled prior to a court hearing. Long delays before disputes get to court, and differences in the quality of the legal advice sometimes available to the parties, can make for unequal contests in a court arena. In the UK and Commonwealth, there is growing concern that the Bolam test is too heavily weighted in favour of a medically countenanced view of what is reasonable care in the circumstances.[33–35] Courts may be too easily swayed by "bottom-of-the-barrel Bolam boys", expert witnesses prepared to testify that:

> practice of a very low order would be regarded as acceptable by a reputable section of the profession. Few of these experts would claim that they themselves advocate or adopt such practice; merely that it is (regrettably) within the range of accepted practice.[4]

Conclusion

An increasingly litigious culture runs the risk of displacing trust and cooperation between doctors and patients with mutual suspicion and defensive professional postures. Although, as the defence societies never tire of telling us, risk management can help minimise negligent conduct,[36] many legal actions arise wholly or mainly as a result of patients simply wanting to tell a story that has not been adequately heard. Allowing time in consultations to listen to the tales of wounded storytellers offers opportunities to reinterpret the relevant patient–doctor encounters, to reconsider what was said or perhaps left unsaid, to recollect actions taken and not taken. Sharing the upset and the disappointment may help to attenuate reflex resort to legal action.

Some such tales that we will hear in the course of our practice will no doubt be the result of negligence that demands and deserves compensation within the present legal framework; other such tales may not. Either way, listening attentively to the tales of injured patients will help reconstruct the medical events that have unfolded, identify deficiencies in health care, fill in missing elements, repair misunderstandings, and help the wounded storyteller to make wise choices when considering whether or not to commence legal action.

Acknowledgment

Though I alone am responsible for the overall interpretation of this chapter, I would like to thank several colleagues, including Brian Leveson QC, Dr John Launer, Dr Paquita de Zulueta, Dr Trisha Greenhalgh and Dr Ruth Richardson, for commenting upon earlier drafts.

1 Frank AW. *The wounded storyteller: body, illness, and ethics.* Chicago: University of Chicago Press, 1995.
2 Stanton S. What really happened to my baby? *Sacramento* Bee November 1993. Quoted In: Gilbert SM. *Wrongful death.* New York: WW Norton, 1997.
3 Hurwitz B. *Clinical guidelines and the law: negligence, discretion and judgment.* Abingdon, Oxon: Radcliffe Medical Press, 1998, pp. 36–42.
4 Irwin S, Fazan C, Allfrey R. *Medical negligence litigation: a practitioner's guide.* London: Legal Action Group, 1995, pp. 1–2, 183.
5 Lord Woolf. *Medical negligence litigation: consultation paper.* Parts 1 & 2. Manuscript, London, 1995.
6 Medical Protection Society. *Information for members: guidance for good practice.* London: Medical Protection Society, undated.
7 Gilbert SM. *Wrongful death.* New York: WW Norton, 1997, p. 43.
8 Czarniawska B. *A narrative approach to organization studies.* London: Sage, 1998.
9 Klinck DR. *The word of the law.* Ottawa: Carleton University Press, 1992; p. 293.
10 Medical Protection Society. Facing the facts. In: *1997 Review.* London: Medical Protection Society 1998, pp. 6–7.

11 *R v Bateman*. Quoted in: Kennedy I, Grubb A. *Medical Law. Text and Materials.* London: Butterworths, 1994, p. 400.

12 *Bolam v Friern Hospital Management Committee.* 1957 2 *All England Reports,* 118–28 at 122.

13 Lord Scarman. Law and medical practice. In: Byrne P ed. *Medicine in contemporary society.* London: King Edward's Hospital Fund for London, 1987, p. 132.

14 Hurwitz B. *Clinical guidelines and the law: negligence, discretion and judgment.* Abingdon, Oxon: Radcliffe Medical Press, 1998, pp. 42–51.

15 *Bolam v Friern Hospital Management Committee.* 1957 2 *All England Reports,* 118–28.

16 Kennedy I, Grubb A. *Medical Law. Text and Materials.* London: Butterworths, 1989, pp. 426–46.

17 *Cork v Kirby Maclean Ltd* (Court of Appeal 1952). *Weekly Notes* 231.

18 *Bolitho v City & Hackney Health Authority.* 1997 3 *Weekly Law Reports,* 1151–61.

19 *Early v Newham Health Authority.* 1994 5 *Medical Law Review,* 215–17.

20 Klinck DR. *The word of the law.* Ottawa: Carleton University Press, 1992.

21 Fleming JG. *An introduction to the law of torts.* Oxford: Oxford University Press, 1985.

22 *Crawford v Board of Governors of Charing Cross Hospital* (Court of Appeal). *The Times,* 23 April and 8 December 1953.

23 *Crawford v Board of Governors of Charing Cross Hospital* (Court of Appeal). In: Mason J, McCall Smith RA eds *Law and Medical Ethics.* London: Butterworths, 1991, p. 211.

24 *Vernon v Bloomsbury Health Authority.* 1995 6 *Medical Law Reports,* 297–310.

25 Goodrich P. *Languages of law.* London: Weidenfeld and Nicolson, 1990.

26 Goodrich P. *Languages of law.* London: Weidenfeld and Nicolson, 1990, pp. 1–11.

27 Dyer C. Justice on the never never. *The Guardian,* 17 October 1997.

28 Medical Protection Society. Facing the facts. In: *1997 Review.* London: Medical Protection Society, 1998, pp. 6–7.

29 Lord Woolf. *Medical negligence litigation: consultation paper,* Part 1. Manuscript, London, 1995.

30 Myers AR. "Lumping it": the hidden denominator of the medical malpractice crisis. *Am J Pub Hlth* 1987; 77: 154–8.

31 Localio AR, Lawthers AG, Brennan TA, Laird NM, Herbert LE, Peterson LM, Newhouse JP, Weiler PC, Hiatt HH. Relation between malpractice claims and adverse events due to negligence. *New Engl J Med* 1991; 325: 245–51.

32 Vincent C, Taylor-Adams S, Stanhope N. Framework for analysing risk and safety in clinical medicine. *Br Med J* 1998; 316: 1154–7.

33 Kennedy I. Negligence: breach of duty: responsible body of opinion. 1995 3 *Medical Law Review,* 195–8.

34 *Albrighton v Royal Prince Alfred Hospital* (1980) 2 *NSWLR* 542 (CA), 562. Quoted in: Kirby M. Patients' rights – why the Australian courts have rejected "Bolam". *J Med Ethics* 1995; 21: 5–8.

35 Kirby M. Patients' rights – why the Australian courts have rejected "Bolam". *J Med Ethics* 1995; 21: 5–8.

36 Medical Protection Society. *Information for members: guidance for good practice.* Medical Protection Society, London, undated.

24 Narrative based medicine in an evidence based world

Trisha Greenhalgh

> A distinction must be drawn between questions of the kind
> science can answer and questions belonging to some other
> world of discourse, to which we must turn instead if they are
> to be answered at all.
>
> *Sir Peter Medawar*[1]

Is evidence based medicine "old hat"?

The two editors of this book, together with many of the chapter
authors, have previously published articles in support of evidence
based medicine, of which a popular definition is "the conscientious, judicious and explicit use of current best evidence in
making decisions about the care of individual patients".[2] "Evidence" in this context is generally taken to mean evidence about
risk and probability derived from research studies on population
samples. It relates especially (but not exclusively) to the results of
randomised controlled trials and large cohort studies, which are
promoted as more valid and reliable than anecdotal reports,[3] a
stance we have supported in the past.[4] Is this book a spoof, or a sell-
out to a new set of values?

Speaking for myself, the answer to both these questions is an
emphatic no. I hope, in this chapter, to convince you that
appreciating the narrative nature of illness experience and the
intuitive and subjective aspects of clinical competence does not
require the practitioner to reject one iota of the principles of clinical
epidemiology. Nor does such an approach demand an inversion of
the hierarchy of evidence so that personal anecdote necessarily
carries more weight in decision making than the randomised

controlled trial. I will argue, furthermore, that genuine evidence based practice actually *presupposes* an interpretive paradigm within which the patient experiences illness and the clinician–patient encounter is enacted.

The limits of objectivity in clinical method

According to the philosopher Karl Popper, science is concerned with the formulation and attempted falsification of *hypotheses* using reproducible methods that allow the construction of generalisable statements about how the universe behaves.[5] Conventional medical training teaches students to view medicine as a science and the doctor as an impartial investigator who builds differential diagnoses like scientific theories and excludes competing possibilities in a manner akin to the falsification of hypotheses.[6] Such an approach assumes the *positivist* paradigm – that there exists an external reality separate from the observer and mode of observation whose properties can be determined through measurement and experimentation (*empiricism*), and whose behaviour can subsequently be predicted from laws thus derived.

The medical profession has aspired to an empiricist paradigm for clinical method for more than a century (see Chapter 15). This approach is based on the somewhat tenuous assumption that diagnostic decision making follows an identical protocol to scientific enquiry – in other words, that the discovery of "facts" about the patient's illness is exactly equivalent to the discovery of new scientific truths about the universe. Until fairly recently, the empiricist framework was loosely applied and rarely questioned. But in the last 15 years or so, the pursuit of greater scientific rigour in medicine has evolved into a collaborative international endeavour whose explicit aim is to establish (and publish in accessible form) what has become known as "best evidence" – systematically collected data on the precision and accuracy of clinical assessments and laboratory tests, the power of prognostic markers, and the effectiveness of carefully specified interventions.[7] Furthermore, there has arisen extraordinarily rapidly a culture in which professionals aspire to frame their consideration of patients' problems in terms of hypothesis-driven questions, and reflect critically on their own practice with a view to improving the proportion of it that accords with "best evidence".[3]

It is surely rather ironic that the efforts of the evidence based medicine movement to formalise and improve the use of scientific method in diagnosis and treatment (which has certainly had direct and measurable benefits for patient care) has begun to raise serious theoretical questions about whether clinical method is a science at all. Indeed, this chapter (and, earlier, the germ of this book) began as my personal quest to find what would be "missing" from clinical method if the rules of evidence based practice were applied in their most unadulterated and unforgiving form. To address this fascinating issue we must first distinguish what evidence based practice *is* from what many people assume it to be.

The evidence based approach to clinical decision making is often incorrectly held to rest on the assumption that clinical observation is totally objective and should, like all scientific measurements, be reproducible. Thus (the argument goes), if medical diagnosis is akin to the process of elucidation in the natural sciences, then two doctors faced with the same set of symptoms and signs should come to the same conclusion about what is wrong with the patient (or the same list of everything that *might* be wrong with the patient in the same order of probability). If there is rebound tenderness on the abdomen when I examine the patient, that tenderness should be predictably elicited by any other competent doctor performing the same examination.

Sandra Tannenbaum summarised this view in 1995. "Evidence based medicine", she wrote, "argues for the fundamental separability of expertise from expert and of knowledge from knower, and the distillation of medical truth outside the clinical encounter would seem to allow both buyers and sellers in the health care market to act independently and rationally".[8]

But although many followers of the evidence based medicine movement (including, I suspect, the politicians and administrators involved in the National Institute for Clinical Excellence in the UK and the federal Agency for Health Care Policy in the USA) would applaud this positivist image of evidence based practice, its founding fathers made no such claim to objectivity. Indeed, it was Professor Sackett and his colleagues at McMaster University who demonstrated that whenever the diagnostic acumen of doctors is studied, different clinicians show a singularly unimpressive level of agreement beyond chance.[9] What they did say was that we should acknowledge *and measure* the level of disagreement between different clinicians in different circumstances rather than dismiss it or attribute it to inexperience or incompetence.

Clinical agreement, expressed statistically as the kappa score,[9] is of the order of 50% for routine clinical procedures such as detecting the presence or absence of pulses in the feet, classifying diabetic retinopathy into mild or severe, and assessing the height of the jugular venous pressure. (Incidentally, cardiologists agreed rather more often than this in diagnosing angina from patients' *descriptions* of chest pain, and, in some studies, rather less often in interpreting the abstracted, "hard" reality of ECG tracings.)[9]

Those who have studied the phenomenon of clinical disagreement, as well as those of us who practise medicine in a clinical setting ourselves, know all too well that clinical judgments are usually a far cry from the objective analysis of a set of eminently measurable "facts". As Richard Asher argued in the bygone era of the medical generalist,[10] and Sackett and colleagues have more recently rephrased in the language of evidence based medicine,[11] the "facts" doctors find when examining patients or their test results are pre-shaped by what they expect and hope to find. Pitting oedema, for example, will be more readily detected in a patient who has just mentioned that she ran out of "water tablets" last week than in someone who made no such comment.

In the language of empiricism, such an approach could be interpreted as *ascertainment bias*, but in the language of social constructionism it reflects the notion that even objective facts are theory laden. As Anna Donald suggests in Chapter 2, theory itself can be understood as a kind of deductive narrative that *predicts* the "fact" of pitting oedema, for which the mind is then prepared. (It is also increasingly recognised that even the most rigorous randomised clinical trials and epidemiological studies follow a narrative course that is highly constrained by the political, cultural and ideological context in which they are planned and undertaken,[12] and that the published paper that describes a major research study tells a limited, partisan and reconstructed story, however much the researchers have striven for ice-cold impartiality.)[1][13]

Thus, the evidence itself supports the claim that doctors do not simply assess symptoms and physical signs objectively; they *interpret* them by integrating the formal diagnostic criteria of the suspected disease(s) (i.e. what those diseases are supposed to do in "typical" patients, as described in standard textbooks) with the case-specific features of the patient's individual story, and their own accumulated professional case expertise. Some authors have argued that this professional expertise takes an exclusively narrative form, and is made up of the "illness scripts" of all the patients the physician has ever seen with similar or contrasting stories.[14][15]

There is, however, remarkably little evidence (and much controversy) about the precise nature of professional expertise and clinical reasoning.[14 16 17]

Empiricism versus narrative in diagnosis: evidence versus the interpreted story?

The "new gospel" of evidence based medicine holds that anecdotal experience, the traditional material of medical practice, is, despite its many interesting features recounted by Jane Macnaughton in Chapter 20, unrepresentative of the "typical" case[18 19] and thus a potentially biased influence on decision making.[20] Evidence based decision making involves the somewhat counter-intuitive practice of assessing the current problem in the light of the aggregated results of hundreds or thousands of comparable cases in a distant population, expressed in the language of probability and risk – the stuff of clinical epidemiology[21] and Bayesian statistics.[22]

How, then, can we square the circle of upholding individual narrative in a world where valid and generalisable truths come from population-derived evidence? It seems to me that there is no paradox. In particle physics, the scientific truths (laws) derived from empirical observation about the behaviour of gases fail to hold when applied to single molecules. Similarly (but for different reasons), the "truths" established by the empirical observation of populations in randomised trials and cohort studies cannot be mechanistically applied to individual patients or episodes of illness, whose behaviour is irremediably contextual and (seemingly) idiosyncratic.

In large research trials, the individual trial participant's unique and many-dimensioned experience is expressed as (say) a single dot on a scatter plot, to which we apply mathematical tools to produce a story about the sample as a whole. The *generalisable* truth that we seek to glean from research trials pertains to the sample's (and, it is hoped, the population's) story, not the individual trial participants' stories. But there is a danger of reifying that population story, i.e. of applying what AN Whitehead famously called the fallacy of misplaced concreteness.[23] Stephen Jay Gould expresses this danger when he says (Chapter 3) that we have a tendency to "… view means and medians as hard "realities", and the variation that permits their calculation as a set of transient and imperfect measurements of this hidden essence".

"Misplaced concreteness" is also an apt description of the dissonance that occurs when we try to apply research evidence to clinical practice. Hunter has suggested that the reason why medical practice cannot constitute a science is that medicine lacks rules that can be generally and unconditionally applied to every case, even every case of a single disease.[24] (This is borne out by Tudor Hart's observation that only 10% of patients in primary care have the sort of isolated, uncomplicated form of hypertension that lends itself to management by a standard evidence based guideline.)[25] Hence, although there are certainly "wrong" answers to particular clinical questions, it is often impossible to define a single "right" one. Hunter continues:

> Clinical education is preparation for practical, ethical action: what best to do, how to behave, how to discover enough to warrant taking action, which choice to make on behalf of the patient. [These] choices are governed not by hard and fast rules but by competing maxims. ... As lawyers, literary critics, historians and other students of evidence know well, there is no text that is self-interpreting. As rules, then, these maxims are relentlessly contextual.[24]

The Concise Oxford Dictionary defines a maxim as either "a general truth drawn from science or experience" or "a principle or rule of conduct". Medical training is certainly replete with maxims of various kinds (for example: "testicular tumours spread to the abdominal lymph nodes", "a history of non-febrile seizures is a contra-indication to pertussis vaccination", "a woman has a right to choose", and so on). Whilst some (it is hoped, a growing proportion of) medical maxims are based on sound biological principles or rigorous research findings, others are little more than dogma handed down to generations of medical students or specialists in training.

The question of *how* the clinician draws on different maxims to achieve an appropriate decision in a particular case is one of the great unanswered questions of clinical method. Take, for example, two pieces of advice commonly given to medical students and junior doctors: "neck stiffness is common in non-specific viral illness" and "suspect bacterial meningitis in a patient with neck stiffness". Neither of these statements is false, nor are they directly contradictory. The former is probably derived from observational frequency studies; the latter from an ill-defined fear of negligence action gleaned from medicolegal anecdotes. But we do not know which of these two maxims will pertain to any *individual* patient with neck stiffness. Hunter suggests that the process of considering successive sets of competing maxims and drawing lessons relevant to an individual clinical case is a perfectly rational process, but not one that can be derived from epidemiological "laws".

Integrated diagnostic judgments: evidence framed within the interpreted story

Box 24.1 shows a comment by a general practitioner in Cardiff cited by Professor Nigel Stott in a lecture on the mysterious nature of general practice, and which I have expanded below into a hypothetical example about Dr Jenkins. Meningococcal meningitis was diagnosed "against the odds" (this GP had seen it only once in 96,000 consultations) on the basis of two very non-specific symptoms and what was, on the face of it, a lucky hunch. Consider the decision sequence in this encounter. Dr Jenkins contemplates the brief history hastily obtained by the receptionist over the telephone and, using his intimate knowledge of the family, begins to put together the story of this illness.

Box 24.1:   Dr Jenkins' hunch

"I got a call from a mother who said her little girl had had diarrhoea and was behaving strangely. I knew the family well, and was sufficiently concerned to break off my Monday morning surgery and visit immediately."

Examples of maxims that might be considered in this case

(a) *We cannot commit ourselves completely and immediately to all patients who seek our help. If we did, we would be swamped, and our overall level of service would suffer.* [61]

(b) *In suspected meningococcal meningitis, the doctor must act urgently with the utmost priority. To do otherwise would be negligent.* [62]

(c) *Diarrhoea in previously well children is generally viral and self limiting.* [63]

(d) *Meningococcal meningitis produces a characteristic rash and neck stiffness.* [64]

(e) *Meningococcal meningitis presents non-specifically in primary care.* [65]

One interpretation of this doctor's action is that he subconsciously compares the script so far with the tens of thousands of "illness scripts" from children who had become (or were perceived to have become) acutely ill over the years, and decides that it doesn't fit with the template "nothing much the matter". The word "strangely" is rarely used by parents to describe the manifestations of non-specific illness in young children (compare, for example, the familiar expressions "off colour", "not herself", "poorly", "washed out", all of which occupy a very different semantic space from the term "strangely").[26] It may be this single word that alerts the doctor to the seriousness of the case.

Of the many medical maxims that come to mind when trying to make sense of this story, Dr Jenkins might take particular note of three (b, d and e in Box 24.1) to inform his decision making. This doctor's skill, which would be exceedingly difficult to measure formally, is to integrate judiciously selected "best evidence" (observational data about the non-specific presentation of early meningococcal disease[65]) with the potential significance of the word "strangely" and his personal knowledge about this family (their uncomplaining track record, the mother's good sense, and the memory of the child as one whose premorbid behaviour was nothing out of the ordinary). Taken alone, neither epidemiological evidence nor the intuitive response to a short but unusual story would have saved this patient, but the integrated application of both has produced a feat we would all be proud to replicate just once in our clinical careers.

Box 24.2 shows the case of Mrs Ahmed, whom I first described in a chapter for a book on evidence based medicine in primary care.[27] Mrs Ahmed's likely condition has been well described anecdotally and explored qualitatively.[28] But epidemiological data on the prognostic accuracy of the patient's interesting set of symptoms simply do not exist, and neither do comparative studies of different management strategies. Mrs Ahmed's GP, Dr Florey, takes time to listen to her story. She learns a great deal in 15 minutes about the emotional pain of this patient's predicament in her own cultural context. Even though the notion of shame associated with cross-cultural marriage does not accord with Dr Florey's own world view, the use of imagination and a wider knowledge of British Pakistani culture (drawn from books, films, informal conversations and so on) allows her to empathise with the patient and "share the story" (see Chapter 22).

Box 24.2: The case of Mrs Ahmed, using Pendleton's task-oriented analysis of the general practice consultation adapted by Sullivan and Macnaughton[66 67]

Task 1
Explore the patient's ideas and concerns about her symptoms

↓

Task 2
Consider the reason for attendance in sufficient detail to reach a diagnosis

↓

Task 3
Review other problems and risk factors

↓

Task 4
Choose an appropriate action for the problem (s)

↓

Task 5
Ensure mutual understanding between doctor and patient and acceptance of further action

↓

Task 6
Establish and maintain a therapeutic relationship with the patient

Mrs Ahmed, a 53-year-old Punjabi woman with no previous medical history, presents with a feeling of sinking in the chest which she attributes to weakness in the heart.

A detailed history does not suggest serious cardiac pathology. Clinical examination is normal. Mrs Ahmed's daughter has recently announced that she intends to marry a man from a different ethnic group, an act that would bring shame on the family. The likely diagnosis is "sinking heart syndrome", an expression of psychological distress and cultural shame in certain Punjabi groups.[28]

The doctor notes incidentally that Mrs Ahmed looks overweight, had high blood pressure recorded recently, and has a strong family history of diabetes.

An ECG is ordered to reassure Mrs Ahmed, even though its sensitivity in distinguishing cardiac from non-specific chest pain is acknowledged to be poor.[29] Practice based counselling is offered but is politely declined. The doctor defers offering dietary advice and diabetes screening at this stage.

The doctor acknowledges, and offers empathy with, Mrs Ahmed's cultural shame. She gives a holistic explanation of the symptoms and reassures the patient that her heart is normal.

The doctor asks Mrs Ahmed to come for a check-up in a month, and makes a note to address cardiovascular risk at that time, or contact her again if she fails to attend.

Evidence from the research literature is used subtly and skilfully within this multifaceted consultation. Again, there are maxims that appear to compete, such as "the objective value of a resting ECG in excluding organic disease in a patient is low in the absence of specific clinical features[29] and may worsen the problem of somatisation",[30] and "in patients suspected of non-organic chest pain, a full work-up of cardiac investigations can be helpful to both patient and doctor".[31] Dr Florey, wishing to demonstrate her empathy and be seen to be helping in a way appropriate to her standing in the patient's eyes, adopts the latter maxim as the relevant guiding principle in this case. The normal result of this investigation supports the clinical story of "sinking heart" and upholds Dr Florey's message that referral to a cardiologist is unnecessary. The ground has been paved for future consultations to address the patient's emotional experiences rather than pursue the collection of additional spurious tests.

Two other maxims that might be considered in this case are "in patients with several major risk factors for coronary heart disease, preventive advice should be a priority"[32] and "successful health promotion depends on sensitivity to cultural norms and expectations".[28 33] Further investigation and advice on the coronary prevention front is a clear priority for the future, but the use of probing questions about obesity, physical activity and a high fat diet may detract from the intimacy of the shared personal story and make the current consultation evidence-burdened. Dr Florey's action (recording in the notes to address these issues at the next opportunity, and to recall the patient if she fails to reattend) is another demonstration of the successful integration of evidence into the interpreted story of the illness.[34]*

* The story of Mrs Ahmed might be presented in a different form – that of a decision analysis (Thornton JG, Lilford RJ, Johnson N. Decision analysis in medicine. *Br Med J* 1992; **304**: 1099–103). In this approach, quantitative estimates are made not only of "facts" (the pre-test probability of organic illness, the predictive accuracy of investigations, the possible harm from a false positive or false negative result) but also of the patient's values and preferences (for example, her strong desire to have an ECG test) and society's rationing choices (the taxpayer's willingness to fund this investigation rather than some other health option for another patient), and these estimates are expressed as mathematical factors in a probability tree. This complex and highly structured approach, which has been explored in detail by Dowie (Dowie J. "Evidence-based", "cost-effective", and "preference-driven" medicine: decision analysis based medical decision making is the pre-requisite. *J Health Serv Res Policy* 1996; **1**: 104–13), is labour intensive and time consuming, and has not proved popular in practice. But it does illustrate the recognition by the evidence based medicine movement that a new theoretical framework is urgently needed to incorporate a wider narrative into "evidence based" clinical decision making.

Hermeneutics: an analytical framework for diagnosis and intervention

The study of interpretation is known as *hermeneutics*, a term originally used in relation to the analysis of ancient Biblical texts and later extended to include any detailed analysis of written, spoken, depicted or enacted stories. Hermeneutics may thus refer to the study of fictional themes, dreams, perceptions, maps and life histories as well as the experience of illness and the finer points of theology. In a very readable review of the hermeneutics of medicine,[35] the American philosopher Drew Leder argues that even though modern medicine rests on a theoretical foundation provided by empiricist science, it clearly incorporates extra-scientific elements – most notably the professional mastery of practical procedures and the intuitive skills that McWhinney described as the craft of medicine,[36] Hunter (citing Aristotle's *Nicomachean Ethics*) termed *phronesis* or "practical reason" (see Chapter 1),[37] and Tannenbaum extolled in the *New England Journal of Medicine* in an article entitled "What Physicians Know".[16]

In acknowledging the interpretive nature of clinical understanding, we are forced to reject the notion of pure objectivity, for the very existence of interpretive possibilities implies subjectivity, ambiguity, and room for disagreement. But to accept the personal and subjective aspects of clinical judgment does not necessarily equate with relativistic anarchy, since all interpretations of a clinical situation are clearly not equally valid. Hermeneutics, both as developed in the literary world and as applied to the study of clinical encounters, is "a structured discipline with teachable methods, canons of good and bad exegesis, [and] ways of arriving at consensual validation".[35]

The doctor–patient encounter takes place in a highly structured transactional space, in which the behaviour of both parties is determined by socialised expectations. In Leder's view, the "text" that constitutes the diagnostic encounter, and which distinguishes it from other human narratives or modes of communication, is a story about the *person-as-ill*. This, in turn, integrates four separate secondary texts:[38]

- the *experiential* text – the meaning the sufferer assigns to the various symptoms, deliberations and lay consultations in the run-up to the clinical encounter;

- the *narrative* text – what the doctor interprets to be "the problem" from the story the patient tells – the traditional medical history;
- the *physical* or perceptual text – what the doctor gleans from a physical examination of the patient;
- the *instrumental* text (what the blood tests and X-rays "say").

The first of these, the experiential text, includes crucially the "realisation" by the person that he or she *is* ill – in other words, the assignation of *medical* meaning to the symptom narrative as distinct from an interpretation in terms, say, of tiredness, distress, unhappiness or grief.[35 39 40] According to the principle of hermeneutics, in which things acquire meaning by being put into language,[41] the very telling of the experiential text gives the illness a deeper and clearer meaning for the sufferer, especially if the telling is assisted by skilled therapeutic listening.[42] Cancer patient John Diamond describes this vividly:

> I told him [the specialist] the story again from scratch – the aches and pains, the glands, the blood test, the lump. And as I told it in full for the first time, I started to worry. As a medical part-work delivered to my own doctor in instalments it had seemed like no more than a catalogue of vague and differentiated symptoms; as a single story it became something else, something with greater narrative possibilities than a mere swollen gland.[43]

As several authors in this book have demonstrated (see Chapters 6, 8, 10, and 18), and other writers have discussed previously,[35 44 45] telling the story of one's illness often has therapeutic as well as descriptive significance. (This reveals, in passing, another dimension of the study of narrative in evidence based practice: there is no reason why narrative based *therapy* cannot be treated like any other medical intervention and subjected to randomised controlled trials of efficacy in population samples.)

The narrative text, or medical history, is a story with two authors: the patient who tells of the illness experience in his or her own words, and the doctor (or other health professional) who constructs a professional interpretation of this story and records it in the medical record. There is always a mismatch between the experiential text and the narrative text, about which there are numerous anecdotal examples[46 47] and some published qualitative research.[48 49] Both Holmes and Launer in this book discuss the role of the professional therapist in assisting the patient construct and interpret his or her own illness narrative, which may, however, still differ significantly from the therapist's own.

The perceptual text is, perhaps, where the practical reason that eludes logical analysis is most readily demonstrated. As Leder observes: "Just as music is heard differently by the educated listener, so the experienced physician hears the murmur, feels the substernal thrill that is lost to the first-year student".[35] Anna Donald develops this argument in Chapter 2 of this book. The perceptual "knowledge" that distinguishes the competent clinician from the novice or the oaf is a language that is learnt by practical apprenticeship. We may search our textbooks in vain for this elusive professional knowledge, for it "resides in the body".[50]

In Leder's "instrumental text", "machines are employed to co-author a fuller story".[35] The shadow on the chest X-ray of a 19-year old student returning from an overland trip across India may be objectively identical to that of a 56-year-old smoker who has never been out of Sweden. Both may have coughed up blood. But the radiologist who looks at the X-rays "sees" tuberculosis on one and a high probability of cancer on the other. According to Leder, the search for the "objective" analysis of diagnostic tests (looking at an X-ray, for example, without a clinical or social history) is a flight from interpretation, and one that is doomed to fail.

Leder's prediction resonates strongly with the call from evidence based circles for the "truth" of the instrumental text (i.e. diagnostic test results) not to be taken as absolute but to be tempered by a knowledge of the precision and accuracy of these tests (such as the false positive and false negative rates), and for such tests to be used judiciously on the basis of Bayesian pre-test probabilities determined by the history and clinical examination.[51]

Box 24.3 describes in anecdotal form the place of diagnostic testing within the unfolding plot of a complex illness, and illustrates how high-technology tests, even when used appropriately, can be "red herrings". The instrumental text can be mis-read, and clinicians misled.

Leder's analysis of the various narratives in the diagnostic sequence addresses only the first part of the clinical encounter. But there is also a *therapeutic* narrative – the formulation of a plan of what to do next, and the enactment of that narrative.[52] Should the doctor order further tests, treat (if so, with what), refer to a specialist colleague, or watch and wait? The increasing recognition that these decisions should arise out of informed dialogue between

Box 24.3: The diagnostic "plot"

When a 40-year-old man comes to the emergency room slurring his words and "unlike himself", the cause is not immediately clear but, especially because his sister had a stroke at 40, stroke is strongly suspected in his case too. A nuclear magnetic resonance image (MRI) shows an enhancing lesion of the brain, and a neurologist is called. Still, the third-year student assigned to the case, who knows little about neurology but had a cardiologist as his first preceptor, thinks he hears a soft heart murmur different from the innocuous systolic-ejection murmur the resident recorded in the patient's chart. A number of clinical rules may be brought into play: maxims that promote scepticism about the family history even as it is kept in mind as a major guidepost, maxims that encourage a review of systems despite the likelihood of stroke. Epistemological maxims, too, may help the student weigh the relative importance of anecdotes, the reliability of both the MRI as a test specific for stroke and the student's own novice perceptions; even the zebra rule ("when you hear hoofbeats, don't think zebras") may be involved. The hoofbeats are there, but what do they mean? Is the student's understanding of the case science? Art? He documents a grade 2 murmur, his working hypothesis is that the lesion is not a stroke but the result of an infection that has seeded from heart to brain. When, soon after, the patient develops a fever, a wholesale interpretation of the case takes place. The student's observation is highlighted, the patient is sent for an echocardiogram, and the diagnosis of endocarditis is made and treatment quickly begun.

In the study of literature, such a development over time is described as plot, and the outline of that plot, its limits, and the expectations that an audience brings to its perception and interpretation are all more or less implied in the reader's recognition of its genre. This case begins with mental status changes, but the story that unfolds is deceptive; the family history is a false lead and even the MRI is something of a red herring. The "real" plot will not be clear until it has unfolded a bit further: we need more time, more clues, a rival interpretation. We get into the bargain an interpreter who is young, skilled, and lucky in his partial ignorance. Is it a cerebral haemorrhage as the signs strongly indicate or, as yet unsuspected by anyone but the third-year student, is it a vegetation that has spread to the brain from the slightly noisy heart valve? This is the case based suspense of clinical medicine. In the interpretative, plot-reading effort that constitutes diagnosis, competing maxims govern the process of fitting symptoms to the disease taxonomy and then determining how best to treat the patient.[24]

Reproduced with kind permission from the author and Kluwer Academic Publishers; see Reference 24.

doctor and patient[53] has revealed a need for further research into the narrative of shared decision making[54] – an aspect of narrative analysis in medicine that will no doubt expand over the next few years.

Conclusion: evidence based practice in a narrative interpretive world

In a widely quoted riposte to the critics who accused them of naïve empiricism, Sackett and colleagues claimed in 1996,

> The practice of evidence based medicine means *integrating* individual clinical expertise with the best available external clinical evidence. [...] By individual clinical expertise, we mean the proficiency and judgment that individual clinicians acquire through clinical experience and clinical practice.[2]

But these authors did not at that time go on to explore the nature of the paradigm that removes the dissonance between the "science" of objective measurement and the "art" of clinical judgment.

If evidence based practice is concerned with the interpretive act of clinical reasoning rather than simply with the mechanical application of empirically derived scientific truths, where does clinical epidemiology's hierarchy of evidence fit in? In Chapter 10, John Launer comments,

> The story-telling approach may collide rather violently with concepts imported from positivist, "objective" viewpoints. [...] Clinicians who stand at the intersection between the world of stories and the world of categorisation, between the hermeneutic role and the World Health Organization's International Classification of Diseases (ICD-10), may well feel that theirs is an impossible position.

When Marshall Marinker asks, in Chapter 11, "On what plane of the imagination do the changes in Hilda Thomson's joints, the look of anger, her husband's interminable convalescence, and her complaint about society's lack of concern for the 'little man' meet?", he offers the answer "on the plane of the imagination which embraces the concepts of whole-person medicine, [and which] requires from the doctor not only a knowledge of the language and grammar of diseases, but also of human mythology". The results of Hilda Thomson's blood tests for rheumatoid arthritis are as much a part of her illness story as the fact that she experiences her husband as a "little man". An accurate knowledge of the precision of different diagnostic tests in populations with joint pain can and should be integrated into the reasoning process.

As Kuhn perceptively predicted,[55] no paradigm can be understood through any other. Indeed, any attempt to do so will tend to generate heat rather than light[56] and leave all parties dissatisfied – after all, how many would agree that "partial narrativism" is the compromise we should all be aspiring to (see Chapter 18)? The empiricist paradigm manifestly fails to encompass the significance of the "little man", and the extreme post-empiricist paradigm refuses to recognise the external and reproducible "truth" of "best [empirical] evidence". But in reality, both clinicians and patients readily transfer between different paradigms even when addressing a single clinical problem.[57]

Because of the interpretive nature of human understanding, the experienced clinician can integrate Hilda Thomson's blood test results with all the other disparate aspects of her personal story which, on a purely logical level, defy taxonomy. Indeed, the results of the blood tests presented in the absence of additional information become impoverished abstractions from which only bland generalisations are possible. They acquire meaning and the legitimacy to influence decision making only when interpreted in the light of Hilda Thomson's unique story.

Similarly, to take a whole-person (or, in this case, whole-family) approach to the "hyperactive" child, Sheryl, described by John Launer in Chapter 10 does not require the doctor to dismiss or ignore the research evidence on drug treatment of attention deficit-hyperactivity disorder. Rather, it requires him to interpret the evidence in the light of this complex story whose strands have been woven in "a matrix of genetics, family and social influences, together with moral choices and fate".

Health professionals, perhaps especially those in primary care, frequently experience frustration when trying to apply "evidence based" research findings to real-life case scenarios.[58-60] I would suggest that this occurs most commonly when they abandon the interpretive framework and attempt to get by on "evidence" alone, as might have occurred if Marinker had suspended his clinical judgment and attempted studiously to follow a "guideline" on the management of seropositive rheumatoid arthritis. The irrevocably case based (i.e. narrative based) nature of clinical wisdom is precisely what enables us to contextualise and individualise the problem before us.[34] [67] Far from obviating the need for subjectivity in the clinical encounter, the valid application of empirical evidence *requires* a solid grounding in the narrative based world.

Acknowledgment

I thank many colleagues who commented on earlier drafts of this chapter, and in particular Dr Brian Hurwitz and Dr JA Muir Gray CBE. The views expressed are mine alone.

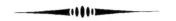

1 Medawar P. *The limits of science.* Oxford: Oxford University Press, 1984.
2 Sackett DL, Rosenberg WMC, Gray JAM, Haynes RB, Richardson WS. Evidence-based medicine: what it is and what it isn't. *Br Med J* 1996; **312**: 71–2.
3 Sackett DL, Richardson WS, Rosenberg W, Haynes RB. *Evidence-based medicine: how to practice and teach EBM.* London: Churchill Livingstone, 1997.
4 Greenhalgh T. *How to read a paper: the basics of evidence-based medicine.* London: BMJ Publications, 1997.
5 Popper K. *Conjectures and refutations: the growth of scientific knowledge.* New York: Routledge and Kegan Paul, 1963.
6 Wulff HR. The foundation of clinical decisions. In: *Rational diagnosis and treatment: an introduction to clinical decision making.* 2nd edition. Oxford: Blackwell Scientific Publications, 1981, pp. 5–17.
7 Chalmers I, Sackett D, Silagy C. The Cochrane Collaboration. In: Maynard A, Chalmers I eds. *Non-random reflections on health services research.* London: BMJ Publishing Group, 1997, pp. 231–9.
8 Tannenbaum S. Getting there from here: evidentiary quandaries of the US outcomes movement. *J Eval Clin Pract* 1995; **1**: 97–103.
9 Sackett DL, Haynes RB, Guyatt GH, Tugwell P. *Clinical epidemiology – a basic science for clinical medicine.* London: Little, Brown & Co., 1991, pp. 19–35.
10 Asher R. *Talking Sense.* London: Churchill Livingstone, 1986.
11 Sackett DL, Haynes RB, Guyatt GH, Tugwell P. *Clinical epidemiology – a basic science for clinical medicine.* London: Little, Brown & Co., 1991, pp. 35–9.
12 Hart JT. Response rates in south Wales 1950–96: changing requirements for mass participation in research. In: Maynard A, Chalmers I eds. *Non-random reflections on health services research.* London: BMJ Publishing Group, 1997, pp. 31–57.
13 Landau M. Human evolution as narrative. *Am Sci* 1984; **2**: 262–8.
14 Schmidt HG, Norman GR, Boshuizen HPA. A cognitive perspective on medical expertise: theory and implications. *Academic Medicine* 1990; **65**: 611–21.
15 Custers EJ, Boshuizen HP, Schmidt HG. The influence of medical expertise, case typicality, and illness script component on case processing and disease probability estimates. *Mem Cogn* 1996; **24**: 384–99.
16 Tannenbaum SJ. What physicians know. *N Engl J Med* 1993; **329**: 1268–71.
17 Sheldon M, Brooke J, Rector A eds. *Decision-making in general practice.* London: MacMillan Press, 1985.
18 Kahneman D, Slovic P, Tverskey A. *judgment under uncertainty: heuristics and biases.* Cambridge: Cambridge University Press, 1982.

19 Plous S. *The psychology of judgment and decision making.* New York: McGraw-Hill, 1993.

20 Dawson NV, Arkes HR. Systematic errors in medical decision making: judgment limitations. *Med Decision Making* 1987; **2**: 183–7.

21 Sackett DL, Haynes RB, Guyatt GH, Tugwell P. *Clinical epidemiology – a basic science for clinical medicine.* London: Little, Brown & Co., 1991.

22 Freedman L. Bayesian statistical methods. *Br Med J* 1996; **313**: 569–70.

23 Whitehead AN. *Science and the modern world.* New York: The Free Press, 1925.

24 Hunter K. "Don't think zebras": uncertainty, interpretation, and the place of paradox in clinical education. *Theoretical Medicine* 1996; **17**: 225–41.

25 Tudor Hart JT. Hypertension guidelines: other diseases complicate management. *Br Med J* 1993; **306**: 1337.

26 Osgood C, May WH, Murray S. *Cross-cultural universals of affective meaning.* In: May WH, Miron SM eds. Urban, IL: University of Illinois Press, 1975.

27 Greenhalgh T, Young G. Applying the evidence with patients. In: Haines A, Silagy C eds. *Evidence-based practice – a guide for primary care.* London: BMJ Publications, 1998.

28 Krause I-B. Sinking heart – a Punjabi communication of distress. *Soc Sci Med* 1989; **29**: 563–75.

29 Pozen MW, D'Agostino RB, Selker HP *et al.* A predictive instrument to improve coronary care unit admission practices in acute ischaemic heart disease. *N Engl J Med* 1984; **310**: 1273–82.

30 Tate P. *The doctor's communication handbook.* Oxford: Radcliffe Medical Press, 1995, pp. 90–5.

31 Baldi F, Ferrarini F. Non-cardiac chest pain: a real clinical problem. *Eur J Gastroenterol Hepatol* 1995; **7**: 1136–40.

32 Lawrence M, Neil A, Fowler G, Mant D. *Prevention of cardiovascular disease: an evidence-based approach.* Oxford: Oxford University Press, 1996.

33 Douglas M. *Natural symbols – explorations in cosmology.* Penguin: London, 1973.

34 Greenhalgh T. "Is my practice evidence-based?". *Br Med J* 1996; **313**: 957–8.

35 Leder D. Clinical interpretation: the hermeneutics of medicine. *Theor Med* 1990; **11**: 9–24.

36 McWhinney IR. Medical knowledge and the rise of technology. *J Med Philos* 1978; **3**: 293–304.

37 Hunter KM. Narrative, literature, and the clinical exercise of practical reason. *J Med Philos* 1996; **21**: 303–20.

38 Daniel S. The patient as text: a model of clinical hermeneutics. *Theor Med* 1986; **7**: 195–210.

39 Heath I. Nature of Medicine. In: *The mystery of general practice.* London: Nuffield Provincial Hospitals Trust, 1995, pp. 17–21.

40 Helman CG. Disease versus illness in general practice. *J Roy Coll Gen Pract* 1981; **31**: 548–52.

41 Rorty R. The contingency of language. In: Goodman RB ed. *Pragmatism – a contemporary reader.* London: Routeledge, 1995.

42 Williams G, Wood P. Common-sense beliefs about illness: a mediating role for the doctor. *Lancet* 1986; **ii**: 1435–7.

43 Diamond J. *C: because cowards get cancer too.* London: Vermillion Books, 1998, p. 21.

44 Scarry E. *The body in pain.* Oxford: Oxford University Press, 1985.

45 Kleinman A. *The illness narratives: suffering, healing, and the human condition.* New York: Basic Books, 1988.

46 Ventres WB. Hearing the patient's story: exploring physician–patient communication using narrative case reports. *Fam Pract Res J* 1994; **14**: 139–47.

47 Marcus L, Marcus A. "Cross-cultural medicine" decoded: learning about "us" in the act of learning about "them". *Fam Med* 1988; **20**: 449–57.

48 Stein HF. The case study method as a means of teaching significant context in family medicine. *Fam Med* 1983; **15**: 163–7.

49 Helman C. The explanatory model. In *Culture, health and illness*, 3rd edition. Oxford: Butterworth-Heinemann, 1994, pp. 111–14.

50 Merleau-Ponty M. *Phenomenonology of perception*. London and Henley: Routledge and Kegan Paul, 1962.

51 Sackett DL, Haynes RB, Guyatt GH, Tugwell P. *Clinical epidemiology – a basic science for clinical medicine*. London: Little, Brown & Co., 1991, pp. 69–152.

52 Mattingly C. The concept of therapeutic emplotment. *Soc Sci Med* 1994; **34**: 811–22.

53 Stewart M, Brown JB, Dorner A, Weston WW *et al*. *Patient centred medicine: Transforming the clinical method*. Thousand Oaks, California Sage Publications, 1995.

54 Elwyn GJ. *Shared decision making in primary care*. Cardiff: Welsh Office, 1997.

55 Kuhn TS. *The structure of scientific revolutions*. Chicago: University of Chicago Press, 1962.

56 Hodgkin P. Medicine, postmodernism and the end of certainty. *Br Med J* 1996; **313**: 1568–9.

57 Rogers S. *Explaining health and illness: an exploration of diversity*. Hemel Hempstead: Harvester Wheatsheaf, 1991.

58 Grimley Evans J. Evidence-based and evidence biased medicine. *Age Ageing* 1995; **25**: 461–4.

59 Asch DA. Why some health policies don't make sense at the bedside. *Ann Int Med* 1995; **122**: 846–50.

60 Greenhalgh T. Evidence-based medicine. In: Hall M, Dwyer D, Lewis T eds. *GP Training Handbook*, 3rd edition. Oxford: Blackwell Scientific Publications, 1998.

61 Tate P. *The doctor's communication handbook*. Oxford: Radcliffe Medical Press, 1995, p. 37.

62 Strang JR, Pugh EJ. Meningococcal infections: reducing the case fatality rate by giving penicillin before admission to hospital. *Br Med J* 1992; **305**: 141–3.

63 Modell M, Mugahl Z, Boyd R. *Paediatric problems in general practice*, 3rd edition. Oxford: Oxford University Press, 1996.

64 Cartwright K ed. *Meningococal disease*. Chichester: John Wiley, 1995.

65 Granier S, Owen P, Stott NCH. Recognising meningococcal disease: the case for further research in primary care. *Brit J Gen Pract* 1998; **48**: 1167–71.

66 Pendleton D, Schofield T, Take P, Havelock P. *The consultation: an approach to learning and teaching*. Oxford: Oxford University Press, 1987.

67 Sullivan FM, Macnaughton J. Evidence in consultations: interpreted and individualised. *Lancet* 1996; **348**: 941–3.

25   Organ music

Ruth Richardson

I have been conducting enquiries in the medical Museum for the past 150 years or so, using what nowadays seems to be the standard interview technique of modern oral historians and ethnographers. Of course, most interviews were undertaken long before tape-recorders were invented, so I have only handwritten notes of past conversations. Looking back over them, I notice that they sometimes include shorthand marks whose full meaning I can now no longer recall – memory does tend to give way after a century or so. Occasionally, too, bindings have perished, or the edges of pages have been nibbled away by mice or bookworms, or even stained with the liquids used in the prosector's office for preserving wet specimens. I realise too with great sadness that – having always been rather impecunious – the paper of which the notebooks were made was not of the best. This being so, many parts of my manuscripts are browned and even flaking with age. Others are bleached or stained, and in some places missing altogether. Moreover, I am no longer certain if the locations of the specimens remains the same now as when I did the work – several wars having supervened, and much recent uncertainty and upheaval besides. This preamble is offered by way of soliciting indulgence for the fragmentary nature of the notes which follow.

My first case report was, naturally, my own. I am the lady many call Mrs Paget, standing in the glass case by the door, bent double by the disease which wedded itself to my skeleton. I was for many years the old Professor's cleaning lady. You would not dream, when looking at my bent-over spine, that I was a fine dancer in my youth. But never mind, I was also a fine cleaner in my maturity. When one's head is fixed so firmly in a downward-looking position one can be extremely attentive to all the nooks and crannies of the Museum floor. I was less apt with shelves, but I did my best.

The Professor appreciated me, and I cared for his precious specimens. I polished their bottles and jars and cases tenderly for many years. And knowing them so well, for so long, was how I came to hear their music.

Ultimately, I decided that since my Professor cared so much for the anatomically curious and the pathologically peculiar, that he and his students should be the final beneficiaries of my affliction. Relieved of my prison, I am now tall as ever I was in my prime. When our string-quartet plays on autumn evenings I dance with all the old gaiety, and not a little added joy.

I am one of the very few in here who knowingly gave their parts to the Museum. If you were to go only by the official catalogue, you would be unaware that most of the parts on show in the glass bottles and cases appear here not as gifts, but as appropriations. A very great number were excised in surgical operations, or found incidentally during post mortems. There operated a sort of unspoken anatomical *quid pro quo*: surgery with a hope of cure in return for the right to confiscate the physical manifestations of disease or deformity. Consent was not felt to be required. Elaborate respect for squeamishness ensured that any uncomfortable questions patients or relatives may have had remained unspoken.

Many of the larger and older specimens date from a time when nothing but grief was offered in consolation to those whose parts were taken. Their identities were known only to the rough fellows who procured them for the Medical School at great risk, from churchyards near and far from London. And even the body-snatchers sometimes had no knowledge of their names – graves being so fresh as to be unmarked in any way save by flowers and tears.

The prevalence of institutional specimens might lead an attentive visitor to conclude that a number of maladies (such as cancers of the adrenals) caused insanity, or perhaps led to destitution. But this is usually an artefact of organ procurement. Before the Great War there was a group of particularly observant pathologists who, having trained under my Professor, knew the Museum's weaknesses, and resolved to supply them. One served the Metropolitan Asylums Board, and two others covered between them seven workhouse infirmaries. We do have a handful of aristocracy, who arrived via the grave-robbers or the post mortem room, but they are far outnumbered by the rest of us. Here all are equal, for no-one can distinguish a king's cancer from a beggar's.

Of course many *mind* quite fiercely that portions of themselves are here without assent, and would infinitely prefer quiet churchyard rest in kindred company. But we all of us understand our curious importance, and have come to terms with the predicament in which our abstracted parts have involved us. We are more than gratified if the horror of our fate prevents another such.

One day, of course, when the trumpet shall sound, all those parts which are now dried, or bottled, or buried in the museum basement, will burst forth from their cases and find their rightful owners – their identity inhering in their being. But on that great Day I anticipate that I myself shall be rather too busy finding my own lost parts: my umbilicus, lost from a dreadful hernia, placenta (or will that belong with the babe?), my excised papilloma, and so on ... (and I wonder if one is reunited with one's shed teeth and hair?) Anyhow, as I say, I anticipate that I shall then be so preoccupied with the novelty of the experience as to be quite unable to give proper concentration to the identities coalescing about me. Perhaps this is why I have been concerned to record these findings: so that until that time we may have at least *some* inkling as to who is whom in this Museum.

Take, for example, the fatty liver in Gallery two, whose lower lobe looks rather as if it were a map of Africa. This particular liver belongs to a rather fine looking woman from the Ball's Pond Road, who fell ill while expecting her seventh child in 1852 and who died rather rapidly in unhappy circumstances. Her child did not survive, and her husband was not swift enough to refuse a post mortem, so her parts were obtained and bottled here before he knew it. The Hospital undertaker was careful to make the body look presentable, and the poor fellow was so full of sorrow gazing at his wife with their dead infant in her arms as they lay in the deal coffin, that he did not think to look inside the shroud. Late at night, you do occasionally hear her singing lullabies in Gallery two, and glimpse her plaiting her long red hair there.

Alongside that specimen, next to the diagram of how tight-lacing rearranged female innards, you can observe the bisected liver of a Brighton lady of a similar vintage who would insist on wearing the tightest corsets. She achieved her ideal hourglass figure and died. Her sweetheart was a very dapper sort of a chap who insisted on a similar mate, and paid the price. Beside her on the shelf you will see the tender little liver of a Chingford lad not two years old, split by a blow from his unnatural father in 1910. The childless and the child comfort one another in the night.

The Museum shelves are strongly made. The old glass bottles with their thick wax seals bear ponderously down with their soft contents. Even the more modern plastic boxes are weighty with precious specimens and preserving fluids. But the impression is of lightness. Kidneys, livers, brains, spleens and other parts (often delicately tethered with tiny threads to glass splints so as to preserve the impression of levity) float in clear, opaque or ambered liquids; held in suspension like the pathological processes they exemplify – arrested growths, odourless suppurations, pain benumbed, decay forestalled.

Afflicted and dissected bodies, long disposed-of, are fixed, too, in anatomical wax models. Casts (made first with wax, then metals, and nowadays with plastic) preserve the coral forms of the blood-vessels which served lungs, kidneys and testes, all long-ago dissolved away.

All manifest the skilful labours of the Museum's Technicians: links in a human chain of expertise dating from before the Museum began in the 18th century. Most of them have now passed away. Their mysterious labours in the preserving room, their secret recipes and esoteric knowledge have secured the transient delicacy of our bodily evidences of human infirmity: disclosed their intrinsic character, displayed their essence, fixed them in timelessness.

The voices of these devoted custodians sometimes echo through the Museum's galleries, and blend with those of the Tutors, whose great unwritten corpus of knowledge, evolving over the centuries, has been the means whereby generation following generation has come to perceive – beyond the catalogue's spare notes and the unhappy evidences of human mutability which crowd the shelves – the medical value of this great repository.

Student voices echo here, too: unguarded conversations and startling thoughts, to which (of course) we are privy. For who can witness without pity the inexorable secret causes of mortal conditions, like the bottles in Gallery two where the huge bubbly sponge kidneys of a father and his son sit together on the same shelf? Each died in coma within twenty years of the other, at exactly the same age, after months of breathless weakness. Or the thigh-bone in Gallery six, split to disclose the invasion of the marrow by a proliferation of cancer cells which deprived a much-awaited three-weeks' child of his mother, and her mourning husband of his darling wife. The contiguous father and son, now each to the other restored, often sing duets here on summer evenings. The young mother – who died from the multiple brain haemorrhages of acute leukaemia (diagnosed as pernicious anaemia of pregnancy) – hums sadder melodies.

So too does the smart tailoress whose failing sight was afterwards found to be caused by a pituitary tumour (a soft coffee-coloured egg-sized specimen in Gallery four) which had atrophied her optic nerves and precipitated a dementia so severe that, having become destitute, she was incarcerated at Hanwell asylum, and died there in 1924.

Some of our exhibits, such as the asphyxia series in gallery five, are displayed almost as cautionary tales on the fragility of human existence. Here the tongues and gullets of various individuals are preserved to reveal the simple manner in which vibrant life may be extinguished – a button in a baby's throat, an inhaled orange segment, a grape, a pickled onion, the cap of a pen, a birthday party balloon. Each individual has a tale to tell – of lives cut short without warning, and terrible unresolved griefs.

In other cases, the pathologies which were of interest to my Professor and his forbears and successors did not cause death at all. There's a very witty grandmother in Gallery three whose non-functioning thyroid cancer was of considerable interest, though she died of a ruptured aorta. She has a marvellous laugh, which echoes beautifully among the bottles.

Another dear lady in the lobby case almost as you enter Gallery three found it bizarre to have entered the Hospital for a painful leg and to have emerged for burial minus her tongue. The acute pain in her limb manifested its cause in breathlessness and she expired in casualty from a pulmonary embolus. Her emboli were no great interest to the old hands in the post mortem room, but her goitre was. Her tongue and all its attachments down to the bronchi are bottled up to display the extensive growth which enwrapped them, it is said (in the official catalogue) without inconvenience during life. The woman herself told me she had thought it churlish to trouble the doctor with her embarrassment at being stared at and her sadness at becoming unable to sing her old music hall songs. She had lost her work as a diamond-grader in Hatton Garden in 1882; no longer able to lower her chin, her eyes could not reach the workbench ... not to mention the difficulty of getting clothes to fit over the growth or of locating scarves long enough to obscure it from prying eyes. Now it is laid bare for all to see, and she sings still.

A lively chap plays ragtime accordion here, just as he did in life. He died from abdominal injuries after a dockside accident in 1934. At the post mortem he was found to have a rare encysted subdural haematoma from an old head injury, which his body had itself cordoned off and rendered harmless inside a membrane, years before. The blood clot, its membrane and the part of his skull to which it was attached are to be found in Gallery four. His dance tunes are often accompanied by sympathetic rhythms on the spoons played by a negro sailor whose almost unrecognizable great foot is bottled up just outside gallery seven to illustrate the distensions and deformities of elephantiasis. He had married a tobacco sorter after jumping ship, fathered two children, and died at Wapping in 1912.

Of course some of us are here because we typify the limits of medical intervention, like the series of white concertinas of synthetic replacement blood vessels and early heart valves blocked with purple blood clots in Gallery five. Or the right kidney of a girl knocked down by a new motor omnibus, who was found after death to have been born without the other kidney the surgeon had expected to be there. Or again, the terrible malignant tumour of the nerve sheath preserved in the nervous system collection, which, despite all the aggressive treatments available at the time grew from a small lump on the collar bone of a fine Nightingale nurse in our Hospital, and eventually extended from her ear to her top rib and right across to the tip of her shoulder.

It is natural, I suppose, that grateful patients sing cheerful tunes, like the three happy men who share a shelf in the dermatology corridor by Gallery seven. Each acquired anthrax at work – one was a fur-cutter, another a jobbing plasterer, the last a leather-dresser – and in each case swift excision of the pustules saved their lives. These three have formed themselves into a barbers'-shop-chorus – and raise the spirits of the entire Museum with their gladsome harmonies.

Although (as I have said) most of the Museum's inhabitants are nameless, the complaints embodied in our parts have descriptive titles of the nicest specificity. We have, for example, "nutmeg" and "sponge" livers, "horse-shoe" kidneys and "staghorn" calculi, and the sonorous titles bestowed upon the sad, strangely beautiful monstrous births which float forever in the Lower Gallery: the harlequins, cyclopses and sireniforms, micromelos, thoracopagus, craniopagus, anadidymus. These little creatures (whose perfect tiny hands remain as wrinkled in the preserving fluid as in the womb) call out to me as I pass, their little faces fixed in sadness at the time of birth – two heads on one body, two bodies fused into a single

271

head, and the quieter ones with only a central eye, or a single mis-shapen conjoint lower limb. They speak to me of their own private agony, and of the horror which greeted their arrival in the world.

Their sadness, however, is mitigated by the Museum's careful project of naming and displaying, which somehow offers the reassurance that such aberrations play a part in the great spectrum of Nature's creation. The same is true of all our infirmities. Visitors cannot be unaware that through us, all look towards their own unknown futures. And, at the same time, the pathos of human malformity serves also to reveal the miraculous generality of perfection.

Alongside the fœtal abnormalities, the miscarried babies, and the pitiful mothers whose ruptured wombs orphaned families of children, perhaps the most poignant of the museum's melodies are those of the unwanted and unloved. The dead-before-their-time – aborted fœtuses and strangled infants found decayed in river reaches, in marshes wrapped in cloths or mummified in attics – and those adults who died alone, like the poor recluse whose entire head floats preserved on the large shelves outside the prosector's door, half-devoured by a fungating cancer of the face, or the tramp on Gallery eight who died out under the sky and became a perfect example of adipocere before being found. He has a permanent home at last. Here, these are appreciated for what they are, while what they were undergoes another process. Relieved of her tumour the old lady has become quite sociable again, and the tramp has surprised us all by proving to be an adept on (of all things) the hurdy-gurdy. He takes for a partner the tiny monkey in Gallery one, and for hours they entertain us with their antics!

Now that I have begun to describe the Museum's inhabitants, I find that – far from having too few as I originally thought – I have in fact too many notes. I have barely begun to tell you of our company. I have missed mentioning half the Galleries, and the many life-stories narrated to me. Perhaps some day I shall be persuaded to compose a longer exposition. Or perhaps you may be induced to visit us yourself?

You need only listen, as to a seashell, at the Museum's open door. We have observed that those with hearts have also the attribute of sensitive ears.

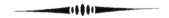

Appendix
Some recommended reading

Trisha Greenhalgh and Brian Hurwitz

Opinion is bound to be divided on which literary works constitute core texts for the student or practitioner of medicine. Literary texts that include medical themes necessarily touch on vulnerability, risk, contingency, disease, disappointment, suffering, and death. The requirements for a "core text", suggests McLellan,[1] include the facility to be read on several levels – literal, symbolic, metaphorical or allegorical. They should tell us something about the practice, history or epistemology of medicine, illuminate the experience of illness, parenthood, disability or "otherness", highlight the importance of cultural factors, or offer insight into the character, education, daily life or decision making skills of medical practitioners.

Woodcock has summarised concisely what the reflective reader can expect to gain from such a text: "sensitivity to complexity of character and situation; heightened awareness of self and other; the ability to embrace contraries and ambiguities and to imagine and empathise with alternative realities; the power to effect catharsis and give meaning; and an appreciation of both the truth-value and the necessary fictionality of the narrative".[2]

Robin Downie adds that literature can give cognitive shaping to the sympathetic imagination, help health professionals come to terms with powerful emotions associated with their involvement with illness and death, and generate (and give meaning to) moral questions about the provision (and withholding) of health care. In addition, Downie adds, many doctors would benefit from the humbling experience of seeing themselves portrayed as figures of fun – pompous, abstruse, self-seeking and avaricious.[3] In a review of how the humanities (philosophy, art, anthropology, law, music, theatre, and so on, as well as literature) might promote *humanity* in the student of medicine, Chris McManus argues that the characters in books, films, and plays act as surrogates for a vast range of real people. He quotes the words of TS Eliot: "we read many books because we cannot know enough people".[4] McLelland's personal choice for core texts in literature for medicine includes *Middlemarch* (George Eliot), *The Death of Ivan Ilyich* (Leo Tolstoy), *The Magic Mountain* (Thomas Mann), *Arrowsmith* (Sinclair Lewis), *The Plague* (Albert Camus), and *Cancer Ward* (Aleksandr Solzhenitsyn). More contemporary titles, suggested in a recent readership poll by the *British Medical Journal*, include *1984* (George Orwell), *The Little Prince* (Antoine de St Exupéry), *To Kill a Mockingbird* (Harper Lee), and *Les Miserables* (Victor Hugo).

The poet and physicaian Danie Abse recommends *The Private Life of Islam* (Ian Young), *Dr Glas* (Hjalmar Soderberg), *Light Up the Cave*, an autobiography by Denise Levertov, and two volumes of poetry, *Beyond Bedlam* (edited by Smith and Sweeney) and *Poems from the Book of Hours* (Rilke).[5]

Grant Gillett, a neurosurgeon and professor of medical ethics, and Barbara Nicholas, a bioethicist, found the following texts helpful in running workshops on narrative ethics for New Zealand doctors: *The Citadel* (AJ Cronin), and *Women Fly When Men Aren't Watching* (Sarah Maitland) – an historical novel recounted through the voice of the woman dwarf upon whom Dr Hugh Chamberlain demonstrated the early use of obstetric forceps.[6]

In Chapter 13 of this book, Steve Rachman suggests, in addition to some of these titles, *Elsie Venner* (Oliver Wendell Holmes), *The Yellow Wallpaper* (Charlotte Perkins Gilman), and the play *The Conduct of Life* (Ralph Waldo Emerson). For an understanding of medical ethics, Anne Hudson Jones (Chapter 21) has suggested, among others, *The Use of Force* (William Carlos Williams), *Brute* (Richard Seltzer), and *Tender is the Night* (F. Scott Fitzgerald).

A number of formal anthologies have been compiled with a view to literature and medicine course work. The On-Line Data Base of Literature and Medicine, maintained through New York University School of Medicine, includes an annotated bibliography of over 800 literary works as well as a selection of medical humanities course syllabi. The internet address of this source is:

http://endeavor.med.nyu.edu/lit-med

Critical understanding of narrative, the ability to appreciate and verify a patient's account, is a core clinical skill (see Chapter 21).

Indeed, it is important to acknowledge that good medical narrative is often to be found in mainstream medical textbooks, and not just in what is classically described as "literature". The textbooks of certain clinical specialties, particularly neurology and psychiatry, discuss especially fascinating stories. A focus upon how distortions of perception and sensation are woven into the narrative of patient experience is found, for example, in Henry Head's majesterial investigations into disturbances in the formulation and expression of language in *Aphasia and kindred disorders of speech* (two volumes, Cambridge University Press, 1926). Volume 2 offers many clinical histories presented in great detail with verbatim dialogue, drawings and the results of ingenious clinical and cognitive assessment tests, many of which have a strong narrative content. (Populist expositions of clinical neurology continue this tradition – see the works of Harold Klawans: *Toscanini's Fumble*, 1988, and *Newton's Madness*, 1990, both published in London by Bodley Head, and the many published works of Oliver Sacks.)

Our personal choice for a selection of literature to enrich and enliven the study of medicine or other health sciences (in addition to the works mentioned above and those extracted elsewhere in this book) is shown below. Note that this list is not intended to be exhaustive, nor do we wish to imply that it is the "best" selection of literature for students of medicine or health care. Rather, it is drawn from the eclectic reading of two practitioners, neither of whom has had any formal training in narrative analysis or followed a special study module or postgraduate degree in literature and medicine.

A Country Doctor's Notebook (Mikhail Bulgakov [translated from the Russian by Michael Glenny]; London: Collins Harvill, 1995). Autobiographical sketches of a newly qualified doctor starting off his career in 1916 as a general practitioner caring for the peasants of rural Russia. His encounters with patients, families, disease, suffering, and the emotional and physical landscape of the community, are portrayed with kaleidoscopic intensity. The author's depiction of his own developing sense of self, and his increasing awareness of the role thrust upon him, makes for gripping reading.

A Fortunate Man: the story of a country doctor (John Berger and Jan Mohr; Penguin Books, 1967). Autobiographical novel of a general practitioner in the 1950s with perceptive reflections on the nature of general practice.

Awakenings (Oliver Sacks; Hamondsworth: Pelican Books, 1976). A book describing the experience of parkinsonism and the hopes and disappointments of a new drug treatment. This book has probably done more than any other in the post-war era to inform the public and health care professions of both the narrative nature, and the humanity, of clinical encounters.

Before I Say Goodbye (Ruth Picardie Penguin 1998). Fleeting last words (collated from her newspaper column, private e-mails, and letters) of a young writer/journalist who died of rapidly progressive breast cancer, aged 32. Includes copies of handwritten notes to her 2-year-old twins.

C: Because Cowards Get Cancer Too (John Diamond; London: Vermillion Books, 1998). Powerful and incisive account by a young British journalist of his smoking-induced throat cancer.

Dr Chekov: A Study In Literature and Medicine (John Coope; London: Cross Publishing, 1998). A new biography which focuses on Chekov as a clinician, epidemiologist and social commentator. As Tudor Hart says in a pithy review, "Chekov lived a short, big, useful life of immense talent and complete integrity, uniting theory with practice."[5]

Frankenstein (Mary Shelley; first published anonymously in 1818 republished by Penguin 1992). A haunting story that reverberates more and more powerfully as we speed towards the next century. Mary Shelley set out to 'speak to the mysterious fears of our nature and awaken a thrilling horror'. The book recounts how Dr Frankenstein animated a corpse he had assembled out of body parts taken from charnel-houses and dissecting rooms. The resulting unnamed creature escapes and wanders the earth, filled with complex emotion, finally wreaking destruction upon its creator and his world.

Illness as Metaphor (Susan Sontag; London: Allen Lane, 1979). The author contrasts the culture bound images and fantasies that have attached to tuberculosis with those accreted by cancer; she finds a matrix of illness meanings at the cultural point where nature, personal experience, literature, and social structure all intersect.

Letter to Daniel: Dispatches from the heart (Fergal Keene; London: Penguin Books, 1996). Collection of pieces from a BBC foreign correspondent including the eponymous letter to his newborn son in which he contemplates fatherhood and reflects anew on the suffering of children he has seen on his travels in zones of war and famine. Also includes a letter to his father who abandoned his family for alcohol and died alone and in poverty.

Montaillou (Emmanuel Le Roy Laduire; Harmondsworth, Penguin 1980). An intricate reconstruction of the mental, emotional and social world of late thirteenth and fourteenth century French peasants. 'Here surely is the widest-angled, deepest focused, most sharply detailed presentation of village life in the Middle Ages, which has ever been or is ever likely to be proffered'. From Geoffrey Grigson's review in *County Life*.

Oranges Are Not The Only fruit (Jeanette Winterson; London: Grove, 1997). Autobiographical novel about emerging sexuality and repression by a homosexual woman who grew up in a strict Presbyterian adoptive family.

Regeneration (Pat Barker; London: Penguin Books, 1995). Novel based on the work of Dr WHR Rivers, the forward-thinking psychiatrist who treated shell-shocked soldiers, including Wilfred Owen and Siegfried Sassoon, at the famous Craiglockhart Hospital during the first world war. Evocative depiction of the psychological terrors of war and (more generally) post-traumatic stress disorder.

Some Lives! A GP's East End (David Widgery; London: Simon and Schuster Ltd, 1993). Account by a London general practitioner of his life and work in an inner city area with high levels of poverty, deprivation and ethnic mix. Dr Widgery committed suicide soon after the book was published.

The Diving Bell and the Butterfly (Jean-Dominique Bauby; London: Fourth Estate, 1998). An account of the "locked in" state following a severe stroke, painstakingly written by a victim who could communicate only by moving his left eyelid. He died soon after the novel was completed.

The Foot of Clive (John Berger; London, Methuen 1962, republished by Penguin 1970 and by Writers and Readers 1979). A novel located in the bye-gone era of a male surgical ward, where patients once stayed long enough to exchange life stories in their banter. Into this mix of clas and cultural identity is brought a patient requiring emergency surgery who, it slowly emerges, is also a murderer ... .

The Man with a Shattered World (Aleksandr Romanovich Luria; Harmondsworth, Penguin 1972). The chronicle of a professor of neuropsychology who for 26 years attended a man brain injured by a bullet. The book pieces together a remarkable story of disintegration and partial recovery using the patient's own journals and the author's notes of his evolving clinical assessments.

The Healing Arts (Robin Downie (ed.); Oxford: Oxford University Press, 1994). An illustrated anthology of poetry, observations, essays, and evocative excerpts which address biographical, philosophical, literary, and historical realms of medicine and healing.

When a Doctor Hates a Patient (Richard Peschel and Enid Peschel; Berkeley and Los Angeles: University of California Press, 1986). Written by a husband and wife team (one a doctor, the other co-director of the Humanities in the Medicine Unit at Yale), the book offers a collection of parallel vignettes in which the husband-doctor frankly recounts his clinical experiences (in autobiographical sequence) which the wife-scholar then places in a literary context.

Wit and Fizz (Selected works of Ruth Holland; London: BMJ Publications, 1998). Collection of prose and short plays by Ruth Holland, who was the book reviews editor of the *British Medical Journal* until her untimely death in a train crash in 1996. Many short pieces are mildly mocking of the medical profession, while showing an underlying sensitivity to the ambiguities of their role. A good choice for doctors (and doctors-to-be) wishing to respond to Downie's invitation[3] to see themselves portrayed as pompous, abstruse, self-seeking and avaricious.

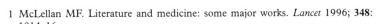

1 McLellan MF. Literature and medicine: some major works. *Lancet* 1996; **348**: 1014–16.
2 Woodcock J (quoted by McLellan, Ref. 1). Teaching literature and medicine: theoretical, curricular and cultural perspectives. In: Clarke B, Aycock W eds *The body and the text: comparative essays in literature and medicine.* Lubbock: Texas Tech University Press, 1990, 41–54.
3 Downie RS. Literature and Medicine. *J Med Ethics* 1991; **17**: 93–8.
4 McManus IC. Humanity and the medical humanities. *Lancet* 1995; **346**: 1143–5.
5 Tudor Hart J. Doctor Chekov: a study in literature and medicine (book review). *Br Med J* 1997; **315**: 1243.
6 Abse D. *More than a green placebo.* Lancet 1998; **351**: 362–4.
7 Nicholas B and Gillett G. Doctors' stories: a narrative approach to teaching medical ethics. *J Med Ethics* 1997; **23**: 295–9.

INDEX